# Hypnotherapy Revealed

THE ERICKSONIAN APPROACH

by Dan Jones

Connect with Dan Jones:
www.YouTube.com/DanJonesHypnosis

Twitter: @AuthorDanJones

First Edition 2018

Published by Dan Jones

Copyright © Dan Jones 2018

Daniel Jones asserts the moral right to be identified as the author of this work

All rights reserved. No part of this publication may be reproduced, stored in a retrieval system, or transmitted, in any form or by any means, electronic, mechanical, photocopying, recording, or otherwise, without the prior written permission of the publishers or author.

ISBN 978- 1728820552

FIRST EDITION

For Abbie

# Hypnotherapy Revealed Series

1. Introduction to Hypnotherapy
2. The Ericksonian Approach
3. Hypnotherapy Trance Scripts
4. Therapeutic Trance-Formation
5. Working with Couples and Families
6. Ideo-Dynamic Healing
7. Hypnotherapy Transcripts
8. Making A Living
9. The Dark Side of Hypnosis
10. Parapsychological Hypnosis

## Contents

*INTRODUCTION* ............................................................. 5

*THE ERICKSONIAN APPROACH* ..................... 9

*FUNDAMENTAL PRINCIPLES* ......................... 35

*PRIMING* .................................................................. 73

*HYPNOTIC LANGUAGE PATTERNS: THE AGREEMENT SET* ............................................. 77

*HYPNOTIC LANGUAGE PATTERNS: LINKING SUGGESTIONS* ................................................... 84

*HYPNOTIC LANGUAGE PATTERNS: PRESUPPOSITIONS* ............................................ 95

*HYPNOTIC LANGUAGE PATTERNS: VAGUE LANGUAGE* ............................................................ 98

*HYPNOTIC LANGUAGE PATTERNS: BINDS* ............. 107

*HYPNOTIC LANGUAGE PATTERNS: COMMANDS & SUGGESTIONS* ................................................ 115

*HYPNOTIC LANGUAGE PATTERNS: METAPHORS* . 123

*PARADOXICAL INTERVENTIONS* ............................. 135

*HOW TO CRAFT HEALING STORIES* ........................ 143

*THERAPY IN ACTION* ................................................ 155

*CONCLUSION* ............................................................ 207

*BIBLIOGRAPHY* ........................................................ 209

Hypnotherapy Revealed

# INTRODUCTION

This book will teach you my perspective of the Ericksonian approach to hypnosis and therapy. It will demonstrate the simplicity that I believe underlies the Ericksonian approach and will teach Ericksonian hypnotic language patterns in a simple and easy to learn and understand way. People often ask whether it is worth taking my online Ericksonian Hypnotherapy training when I say about it being simple and that the hypnotic language patterns are taught in an easy to understand way. They tell me that they had heard it is very complicated to understand and do, I was even told this when I started out as a professional hypnotherapist. I met with experienced hypnotherapists to get advice about setting up in practice and when I said I was learning an Ericksonian approach all the hypnotherapists I met told me "not to bother with that, it is all too complicated, it doesn't make sense. Just start building up a folder of scripts that you can read to clients and stick to these." **This is a myth.** The way I teach is from the principles up, not from the language patterns and techniques down. Teaching it from the principles up means that you will be using all the hypnotic language patterns and techniques automatically and instinctively before you have learned the labels for them consciously so that by the time you are learning them they make sense because you recognise you have been using them already.

On my live training I have people hypnotising each other unscripted using an Ericksonian approach within 30 minutes – **it really is that easy to do** and this gives attendees so much confidence. This often unnerves attendees who have studied hypnotherapy before and only ever used scripts, but for complete beginners who haven't started using scripts as a crutch, this feels such a natural process that they never decide to become script-based hypnotherapists. Hypnotherapy is an unusual therapeutic modality. You don't find counsellors, psychotherapists, youth workers, parenting support staff, educational support staff, social workers, family therapists, addiction counsellors, cognitive-behavioural therapists, psycho-analysts, or any other talking therapies workers feeling the need to do all their work with a script. Yet many hypnotherapists want a script for working with this type of client and a script for working with that type of client, yet they are doing talking therapy the same as all of these other professional's but worryingly don't seem to believe in themselves and their training enough to do the *therapy*.

Although I say I am teaching an Ericksonian approach in this book what I really mean is I am teaching you my perspective on therapy. After more than 20 years doing hypnotherapy I have developed my own views and understandings and had many *a-ha* moments that have shaped my work. Good therapists and trainers who evolve and continually learn and develop end up creating their own unique style. So, for example, hypnotherapy trainer Stephen Brooks (who was the person that first taught Erickson's techniques here in the UK back in the late 1970's) may be thought of as an Ericksonian hypnotherapy trainer but he teaches his evolution of therapy. Ernest Rossi teaches and does his own evolution of therapy, and their versions of therapy today are very much their own approaches, distinct from how they interpreted Milton Erickson's work when they started out, and so it is for me. I have evolved to practice my own approach, but like with Stephen Brooks, Ernest Rossi, or any other well-known Ericksonian hypnotherapist I can't just give my approach a different name like *Jonesian* hypnotherapy because no-one would have heard of it, just like no-one would have heard of *Brooksian* or *Rossian* hypnotherapy. So publicly I just say I do Ericksonian hypnotherapy, but it is important to note here that I don't think of myself as an Ericksonian hypnotherapist, or even a hypnotherapist. I use my interpretation of the Ericksonian approach to underpin how I approach doing therapy, but I think my views of trance and other areas are different to that of Milton Erickson as you will see throughout this series.

In this book I share the skills to use so that you can take the knowledge you have from book one about hypnosis, pattern-matching and the trance nature of reality and use this therapeutically with clients. The knowledge you will gain from this book can be mastered allowing you to be able to confidently hypnotise and therapeutically work with almost anyone using the approach that is right for them as an individual. You will be able to do what I think of as client-centred hypnotherapy.

# The Ericksonian Approach

I often describe myself as employing an Ericksonian approach to therapy. Although I describe myself as that, I don't think of myself as that. I think of myself as someone who does therapy and who tries to take an evidence-based look at the therapy that I do. It is important to me to try things out and find my path, but also, to use what the evidence says is most effective at helping people with different presenting problems and be willing to change what I do and teach in line with evidence, not dogmatically stick to something because I like it. The reason I describe myself as employing an Ericksonian approach to therapy is to associate myself with something familiar to people, so that they have a general idea of how I work or what types of skills I may employ. If I started saying I do a Jonesian approach to therapy, one, it sounds arrogant to me, to name an approach after myself. Even Milton Erickson, who the Ericksonian approach is named after never described himself as doing an Ericksonian approach and who has ever heard of a Jonesian approach to therapy? Would people know what I was talking about? The difficulty is that everyone has a different view of what different approaches mean to them, me included and the public have no idea about many approaches. One of the reasons for writing this book is to explain what I do and don't mean when I talk about the Ericksonian approach.

The shortest answer to what I mean when talking about using an Ericksonian approach, is that *I utilise my observations towards a goal.* Because I utilise my observations I am rarely dictatorial and my therapy can generally look soft and gentle. The only time it isn't soft and gentle is if my observations have led to me taking a different approach in that situation, so, part of the understanding I like people to have of me, is that I practice therapy client-focused, not therapist-focused. I don't try to make clients fit my way of doing therapy, I try to fit their way of doing therapy. This is all fine in relation to other therapists, they may not agree exactly on what they think of when thinking about the Ericksonian approach, but hopefully most think of something which covers these areas. The general public are different as they won't have heard of the Ericksonian approach. I don't like to call myself a hypnotherapist because all therapists do hypnosis, the only difference is that hypnotherapists publicly admit to this and may have had training in hypnosis so that they can do a better job of hypnosis than perhaps a therapist without formal hypnosis training. I am open about the fact I practice hypnosis and that I don't like to call myself a hypnotherapist, but I often end up calling myself a hypnotherapist because it is a term the public have some understanding of and if they have a problem with hypnosis I want to be open about it and let them voice their concerns so that I can talk to them about hypnosis and debunk any myths they may hold.

The difficulty is that many people have a view on what they think a hypnotherapist is and what they do and that all hypnotherapists essentially do the same thing, so it is just a case of going to the cheapest one and you should get the same treatment as if you went to the most expensive therapist. Someone may feel that perhaps the more expensive therapist has more experience or more training, maybe they are better at what they do. In reality you can get rubbish hypnotherapists who charge a lot of money and incredible hypnotherapists who charge very little. Each individual will have their own views about what a hypnotherapist does and what their expectations are about having hypnotherapy. It is common for people to think that the hypnotherapist will command them to *sleep* and will then re-programme their mind, and that during this process they will have no awareness because they will be in a deep trance and afterwards their problem will have gone away. If the hypnotherapy isn't 100% successful in that single session they will conclude they can't be hypnotised and it doesn't work for them. If they remember anything from the session or didn't *feel* hypnotised they will conclude they weren't hypnotised and it isn't any good. In his books and lectures Jeff Zeig talks about finding out from clients what they expect the experience of hypnosis to be like, obviously clarifying any misconceptions the client holds and establishing an agreement of what the experience of being hypnotised will be like and then as a hypnotherapist working towards giving the client the experience they feel would constitute as hypnosis and ratifying this with them as being hypnosis (Zeig, 2014). If a client felt hypnosis would be something deeply relaxing, then the therapist could do a deeply relaxing hypnotic induction, if they felt that they would probably lose awareness of their body, then you could do this as the induction, if they thought they would feel energised, then this would be elicited as part of the induction.

I mention these problems with description of Ericksonian Hypnotherapy because they are both terms linked to me and what I do and terms linked to what I am writing about in this book and yet almost everyone will have their own views of these terms meaning two people could think about Ericksonian Hypnotherapy and both be thinking about something completely different. I have already shared my perspective on hypnosis, on how hypnotherapy is just hypnosis being used in conjunction with some form of therapy, so you get psycho-dynamic hypnotherapists, cognitive hypnotherapists, cognitive-behavioural hypnotherapists, solution-focused hypnotherapists, client-centred hypnotherapists, etc. Some people use multiple therapeutic approaches and may call themselves integrative hypnotherapists, curative hypnotherapists, etc., others may use a label of an approach to hypnotherapy or to convey their training, so you may have Ericksonian hypnotherapists, medical hypnotherapists, clinical hypnotherapists. Then you get people describing themselves by what they focus on treating, like smoking cessation hypnotherapist, gastric band hypnotherapist, weight-loss hypnotherapist, hypnobirthing practitioner. In this section I will cover what I mean when I talk about the Ericksonian approach and what I don't mean, as well as sharing about hypnotic language patterns, therapeutic storytelling, observation skills, paradoxical interventions and what I consider the fundamental principles of the Ericksonian approach.

The Ericksonian approach is named after Milton H Erickson MD. He didn't refer to what he did as being Ericksonian. I think the first record of the term Ericksonian was in a presentation by Jeff Zeig in 1977 (Zeig, 1977). At the time Ericksonian was first used Milton Erickson was still alive. The term was used for the first Ericksonian congress. Erickson died in 1980 before the congress took place, however he seems to have been okay with the term being used, but I don't think he would really have wanted to have thousands of therapists out there claiming to do *his* approach to therapy, when no-one really knew what it was that they were doing and calling Ericksonian because there was nothing written down to define the Ericksonian approach (Lustig, 1988). Some practitioners focused on the therapeutic techniques, others on the hypnotic language patterns, others on aspects of what he did, like focusing on being indirect, using metaphors and stories, or being strategic and some focused on trying to find a therapeutic model or deeper theory behind Erickson's work. Many different approaches to therapy arose or were influenced from therapists studying the work of Erickson, like solution-focused therapies, strategic therapy, family therapy, systems therapy and neurolinguistics programming. Erickson himself often stated "Don't try to imitate my voice, or my cadence. Just discover your own. Develop your own techniques. Be your own natural self." (Parsons-Fein, 2013). He encouraged people to learn different approaches, techniques and theories, to study different subjects like anatomy and anthropology, to develop observation skills, but to then find their own path and develop their own approach.

I feel that many people have over-complicated the Ericksonian approach. That isn't to say that there isn't complexity, just that I feel there is simplicity underlying that complexity. Simplicity also doesn't mean easy. Learning the rules of chess is simple, but that doesn't mean once you know the rules you are a chess master. You have to practice and learn. In chess, you may learn different strategies, different combinations of moves which seem to work well under certain circumstances. As a beginner, you may over-rely on these moves and use them when it would have been best to do something else. As you practice, you get better at seeing the layout of the board and how the game is likely to go over the next few moves, perhaps even having an idea of what moves you may be doing in 10 moves time. With even more practice, you learn to be flexible and start to adapt and change your approach as you get feedback by what your opponent does and eventually you can become very proficient at the game. So, learning the rules of chess is easy, but mastering chess takes focused practice and hard work.

There are many descriptions or definitions of what an Ericksonian approach is. Some people talk about Ericksonian hypnotherapy or Ericksonian hypnosis, others Ericksonian psychotherapy. Some now talk about conversational hypnosis or hypnotherapy or indirect hypnosis or hypnotherapy. Personally, I see indirect hypnosis and conversational hypnosis, etc., as not being an Ericksonian approach, but being approaches inspired by aspects of Erickson's work. Indirect hypnosis is an approach developed by Stephen Brooks and conversational hypnosis was developed by Igor Ledochowski.

## The Ericksonian Approach

Here are some definitions of Ericksonian approach from across the internet:

"Ericksonian hypnotherapy (or indirect, metaphorical hypnosis) is the term used to describe a very specific type of hypnosis which is hallmarked by the use of indirect suggestion, metaphor and storytelling, as opposed to the direct type of suggestion that was its predecessor." Natural Hypnosis (What is Ericksonian Hypnosis and What Characterizes It, n.d.).

"Ericksonian Hypnosis is a method of indirect hypnosis named after Dr. Milton Erickson." British Hypnosis Research (What is Ericksonian Hypnosis? Definition & History, n.d.).

These sites go on to give fuller explanations about Erickson's work and contributions about different techniques he employed and differentiating between Erickson's approach where he would often use an indirect, permissive and conversational approach versus what has become termed traditional hypnotherapy which is usually more direct and formulaic, often using generic scripts and about the hypnotist doing something to a client, rather than evoking something from within a client. Obviously, this is a generalisation and there are times an Ericksonian hypnotherapist will be direct and times a traditional hypnotherapist will be more permissive.

Erickson described hypnosis as "...the communication of ideas and understandings for the purpose of eliciting responsive behavior at both psychological and physiological levels." (Erickson M. H., 1980). And trance as "active unconscious learning" (Erickson & Rossi, 1976). He described what he did as accepting and utilising client's responses, stating "All I know is that they'll respond in an appropriate fashion, in a way which best suits them as an individual. And so I become intrigued with wondering exactly how their unconscious will choose to respond. And so I comfortably await their response, knowing that when it occurs, I can accept and utilize it." (Gilligan, 1982). Talking about therapeutic orientation Erickson said "I invent a new theory and a new approach for each individual." (Lankton & Lankton, 1983).

Erickson used what he felt was right for the client and the situation whether this was direct, indirect, using metaphors or tasks or any other techniques, ideas or approaches. My perspective of an Ericksonian approach isn't about focusing on any of these areas, it isn't about being indirect, Erickson was frequently very direct right through to the end of his life, although it is true he used more indirect techniques than traditional hypnotherapists and he felt that being indirect, gentle and permissive was often the best approach to take where being direct could elicit resistance (Erickson M. H., 1964) (Erickson M. H., 1964). It isn't about always being metaphorical as Erickson often appeared to use stories from his own life, or about nature, or things which were familiar to the client, like talking about baseball and muscle control with a child with an interest in baseball (and who also wet the bed), as a way of teaching them about controlling their bladder and helping them to understand that they have the knowledge, they just need to transfer that knowledge of muscle control to another part of their body (Zeig, 1980). He also set metaphorical tasks like climbing a mountain to think about a relationship (Zeig, 1980), or having a heroin addict search for two identical blades of grass (Rosen, 1991). It is about being client-centred and doing what is right for the client in front of you while authentically being yourself. If the therapist is doing this they will likely naturally be more permissive and use more indirect methods with most clients.

With the focus people often have on certain aspects of the Ericksonian approach and claims that are often made by Ericksonian Hypnotherapists and were made by Erickson himself, it is helpful to explore what research says about various aspects of what most people see as the Ericksonian approach.

In the article *Ericksonian Hypnosis: A Review Of the Empirical Data* (Matthews, Conti, & Starr, 1999) Ericksonian hypnosis is described as having four basic assumptions:

1. Hypnosis is an altered state of consciousness.
2. There are markers of this altered state that distinguish it from the waking state.
3. Hypnotisability of the subject/client is more a function of the hypnotist's skill (i.e. utilization strategies) than the subject/client's ability.
4. The use of indirect hypnotic suggestion is, at least in some instances, more effective in producing hypnotic responses than is direct suggestion.

The research doesn't favour the Ericksonian view of hypnosis outlined with these four points. I will discuss some of the research shortly, but I would disagree with some of these assumptions as being what defines the Ericksonian approach.

The Erickson Foundation defines Ericksonian therapy as "An experiential, phenomenologically based approach to problem solving that utilizes existing client attributes while evoking natural processes of learning and adaptation." (Short, 2017).

I have already shared about Erickson viewing hypnosis as an altered state which differs from the points above and what he meant by that, which differs from the definition used above. In a presentation in 1960 Erickson discussed hypnosis. He shared "I regard hypnotic techniques as essentially no more than a means of asking your subjects (or patients) to pay attention to you so that you can offer them some idea which can initiate them into an activation of their own capacities to behave." He then continued talking about this *special state of awareness or consciousness* which led to him being questioned about his use of these terms, he clarified with "I would like to respond to Dr. Sarbin's comments about an altered state of awareness. If I wanted Dr. Sarbin to say a large number of very pleasant things, I think I would introduce him into a setting where there was soft music and flowers and sufficient other attractions which would induce in him the desire to say a number of nice soft words. However, if I introduced him into a situation where I was tormenting a dog, I expect I could induce him to say a great many unpleasant things. You alter a person's state of awareness by the conditions associated with, and the character of, the stimulation which you offer along with the inner behavior of potentials in that person. I do not think that I am in error to give the general term "state of awareness" to the memories, ideas, and emotions characterizing a person at a given time, nor do I consider this a 'mystical appellation.'" (Erickson M. H., 1980).

Erickson observed that what people could do in hypnosis, could be done outside of hypnosis. The difference was hypnosis helped narrow the client's attention on what is important and just like when you turn down music and stop talking when you try to park a car, you do things better when you pay them your full attention. There may not be any clear sign of an altered state distinguishable from the waking state, but as mentioned earlier in the book, there is evidence of changes in neural activity associated with increased focus of attention, enhanced somatic and emotional control and reduced self-consciousness (Jiang, White, Greicius, Waelde, & Spiegel, 2017) which could be described as an altered or special state of awareness as Erickson described it.

There were areas Erickson was likely wrong. For example, he claimed that hypnotised subjects were more literal than non-hypnotised subjects. Research on literalism in and out of hypnosis has found no evidence of this, so it is likely that Erickson perhaps influenced his own results by knowing what his theories and expectations were (Lynn, et al., 1990).

For point three, that hypnotisability of the client is more a function of the hypnotist's skill (i.e. utilisation strategies) than the client's ability, I would argue that it depends on how you think about utilisation and about hypnosis. I have shared already that I wonder whether what I do is hypnosis or not, because what I would label hypnosis is very broad, so broad that it makes the definition meaningless. I think that hypnotisability is a function of the client's ability rather than a function of the hypnotist's skill. The role of the hypnotherapist is to facilitate the client's innate abilities, to support them in experiencing hypnosis and in the case of therapy, to support them in working towards their therapeutic outcome. The therapist actually does as little as possible.

Erickson described that "hypnosis should primarily be the outcome of a situation in which interpersonal and intrapersonal relationships are developed constructively to serve the purpose of both the hypnotist and the subject...Whatever the part played by the hypnotist may be, the role of the subjects involves the greater amount of active functioning—functioning which derives from the capabilities, learnings, and experiential history of their total personalities. Hypnotists can only guide, direct, supervise, and provide the opportunity for subjects to do the productive work." (Erickson M. H., 1952).

The article gives an example of a story Erickson told about his 3-year-old son Robert falling over and requiring stitches and the intervention which helped Robert through the situation. Erickson directed Roberts' attention to the pain and acknowledged the pain Robert was experiencing, he then directed his attention to the colour of the blood and to counting how many stitches he received. Erickson said that the question could be asked about when hypnosis was employed and stated that "hypnosis began with the first statement to him and became apparent when he gave his full and undivided interested and pleased attention to each of the succeeding events that constituted the medical handling of his problem."

The article uses this as an example of the creative utilisation that Erickson would employ to help bring relief to people but questioned whether this was hypnosis and that it could just have been a distraction technique, that Erickson was more interested in whether an intervention worked rather than how the intervention would be defined. This is an important point in relation to the Ericksonian approach. I wouldn't call it Ericksonian hypnosis, indirect hypnosis or conversational hypnosis. What is important are the Ericksonian principles and although we will cover hypnotic language patterns, it isn't about the hypnotic language or about whether you are doing hypnosis. It is about whether you are doing what is right for your client in that moment, which involves applying your knowledge in a client-focused way.

It could easily be said that what Erickson was doing with Robert isn't hypnosis because if it gets classed as hypnosis, it means almost anything involving guiding and focusing attention is hypnosis. To me, if I had to give it a definition I would say it is hypnosis. It isn't a structured induction to find something to focus on (that spot on the wall for example) and to pay that thing all of your attention (like paying the spot all of your attention) and in doing so, shutting out stimuli that isn't within that focus of attention and then moving this attention elsewhere after beginning to follow the presented ideas (like inside, into thoughts or feelings when suggested). Instead attention is focused on elements of the ongoing experience and directed from one part of the experience to another, narrowing that focus of attention away from other thoughts, feelings and external stimuli towards those aspects of the ongoing experience and at each stage Robert is following the suggestions for where to focus.

The fourth point about the use of indirect suggestions is an interesting one. Research currently seems to point to indirect suggestion being about as effective as direct suggestion, not more effective. There are some circumstances where direct suggestions seem more effective and other times indirect suggestions come out on top, but there isn't much in it between the two. Indirect suggestions may be better at producing post-hypnotic behaviour than direct suggestions, but it seems indirect suggestion is no different than direct suggestion in trying to have success with resistant clients. One of the claims about Ericksonian hypnosis is often that you are indirect to get around or utilise resistance. This is a complex issue. It depends on what is being thought of as resistance. If a client doesn't want to be hypnotised they may well just decide to ignore the suggestions regardless of whether they were given directly or indirectly. If on the other hand, they are given a suggestion to follow and they don't respond to the suggestion despite wanting to, or to be direct could mis-match the client in some way, then I would say that it makes sense to be indirect and being indirect may well work. Currently there isn't research to back this up, so I can only draw upon my own experiences and the experiences of hypnotherapists I know. If I suggest an arm levitation to a client and they want to be hypnotised, they want the levitation to work and their arm just sits on their lap, they may perceive this as failure and this could impact on future successes. It doesn't matter whether they are *in hypnosis* or not according to a hypnotisability scale, their subjective experience would be that it isn't working. If, on the other hand I suggest that they pay attention to their hand and notice what that hand feels like, notice whether it feels heavy or light, warm or cool, etc., then utilised whatever the client told me was happening and fed this back to them to deepen their focus around whatever ideas and experiences they had shared, then there would be no failure, again, this is regardless of whether they would be deemed hypnotised or not according to hypnotisability scales.

Indirect suggestion doesn't make the client more likely to follow the suggestion as is often claimed in courses, where they may state that "because the suggestions are indirect or conversational they go undetected and are followed because the conscious mind hasn't recognised them, so they don't put up resistance."

This type of view is incorrect. It is true that sometimes indirect suggestions may go unrecognised, but the person still has the choice whether they will follow the suggestion or not. About half of subjects may not follow any given suggestion. Obviously, in therapy the client will be more likely to follow suggestions and presented ideas because they are there to get help overcoming a problem and it would be counter-productive to them to not engage with the therapy to some extent, and there is research that unlike indirect suggestions, indirect approaches work – for example, telling a teen to stay awake all night as an indirect approach to getting them to fall asleep. Depending on exactly what the therapist is doing, indirect techniques aren't totally covert. Intelligent and observant subjects can notice or work out what the therapist is doing. Research seems to also point towards clients feeling more resistance towards therapists who use indirect suggestion compared to direct suggestion. This could be because depending on how indirect suggestions are presented they can feel manipulative and like people experience from sales persons who are trying to manipulate them into making an unwanted purchase and doing so indirectly. Whereas using an indirect approach, like presenting a metaphor to help a client with their problem, is often seen as positive and the client feels a sense of trust towards the therapist.

So, objective responses, like the actual depth of hypnosis and responses to suggestions are no different between indirect or direct suggestions, but subjective responses, like how the subject feels and what they think about their experience are different, with a greater number of subjects being more resistant towards the hypnotist when indirect suggestions are used, but possibly also feeling more hypnotised (Matthews, Conti, & Starr, 1999).

Hypnotherapy researchers feel that these areas mentioned above aren't what makes the Ericksonian approach. It isn't the indirect language patterns or the definition and ideas of hypnosis and hypnotisability that Erickson held, what the Ericksonian approach could be understood as is "having the ability to increase client motivation, expectancy and belief that therapeutic change can and will occur." (Matthews, Conti, & Starr, 1999).

To me, the Ericksonian approach isn't a therapy. Milton Erickson had many therapeutic ideas and thoughts based on his knowledge and experience and would develop effective and often creative ways of helping people, but, if you strip back the therapeutic work and strip back the hypnotic interventions, what you find is that underlying it all are some simple fundamental principles. This is what I want to share in the next chapter, it is these fundamental principles which have resulted in so many different styles of the Ericksonian approach. The therapeutic approach which arises is unique to the therapist applying the fundamental principles and their training, knowledge and experience. The Ericksonian approach itself isn't the therapy but the principles therapy is carried out through, or the attitude to therapy as I prefer to think of it.

So, a Jungian analyst could start doing their therapy through the principles of the Ericksonian approach, as could a solution-focused therapist, or cognitive-behavioural therapist, or any other therapist. This way you can see many different therapists doing very different therapy but all using an Ericksonian approach.

I did a job where I had to work in a psychodynamic way, so while I was in that job I took an Ericksonian approach attitude. All documents I had to fill out were completed as per the approach I was using, anyone watching me work would see that I was using a psychodynamic approach to my therapeutic work but underlying it all the time was the

Ericksonian approach. I used to describe that I was *being* Ericksonian. I think of it as something you make a part of who you are rather than something you do. I wasn't *doing* Ericksonian approach, I was *being* Ericksonian. A few years later I was doing a role which required me to do a very different therapeutic approach. I had to use a solution-focused approach. I generally prefer using a solution-focused approach, compared to a psychodynamic approach, but used purely and as it is often taught, can still be restrictive and not as client-centred as I would like, so I used a solution-focused approach to my therapeutic work, but underlying this was the Ericksonian approach. This is what I hope to help you see here, that whatever therapeutic orientation you have it will come with set structures and ways of thinking about things which may have validity in some contexts but may be restrictive in others and becoming client-centred through the development of the Ericksonian approach will help you to expand your hypnosis and therapeutic skills. It can also be applied to other areas of life.

Following the chapter on the fundamental principles of the Ericksonian approach I cover hypnotic language patterns. What I have done with the language patterns is to simplify them by chunking different patterns into categories, so, for example, what I call the agreement set consists of the yes-set and the reverse-yes-set. Linking suggestions consists of compound suggestions and contingent suggestions. There are many books which break down hypnotic language patterns into smaller and smaller chunks. From my years of teaching, what I have found is that when people are presented with vast amounts of information they become overwhelmed and confused. Students and those new to hypnotherapy would focus so much on trying to work out what language patterns they are using and what each pattern is that they would tell me they don't think they are very good because they always forget the different patterns. When I teach hypnosis, thirty minutes into my training I have people hypnotising each other unscripted. Fifteen minutes of that thirty minutes was spent introducing myself and saying what the course will cover, the other fifteen minutes was telling students how to do hypnosis without scripts and doing a demonstration, then I tell them to pair up and get on with it. I don't teach them hypnotic language patterns at this point, I let them do the hypnosis, then during discussion about how they got on I share with them how they will have been intuitively using hypnotic language patterns just because they were using the fundamental principles. I don't want them to have their focus on the language patterns, I want their focus on the client.

This is why I teach in this way. I like to start broadly so that students are hypnotising and using hypnotic language patterns without knowing the names of the patterns or realising they are using them, then, I like to teach them what I would term classes of language patterns, like linking suggestions or the agreement set. This keeps the language pattern learning easy. What I find happens on courses is that once students learn a class of language patterns, like the agreement set, they recognise it as something they were using already. Now they know about that class of language patterns they can practice it and use it more. They don't have to try to learn the names of the different language patterns within that class. This is especially the case with language patterns like double binds. I just teach it as double binds, but there are many types of double binds. When I used to teach each individual language pattern students would lack confidence because they would say they couldn't remember the different binds when they were trying to work with someone. I have known many hypnotherapists who I feel are highly skilled and do a great job, tell me the same thing. That they struggle to remember all the different language patterns and how and when to use them. If the student learns the fundamental principles of the Ericksonian approach they will be using the language patterns automatically. If they learn the classes of language patterns they will be more conscious about the hypnotic language they use and will be using many of the language patterns without knowing the individual names of each pattern. If the student is still interested in knowing more and learning the various language patterns in detail, like the names of the different types of double binds then they can go and do this, but I would recommend doing this after they have made all this prior knowledge instinctive and they understand it all, so that even if they don't remember the name of a specific language pattern, they know this doesn't matter, they are more than confident at using all of the classes of language patterns and the fundamental principles.

# Fundamental Principles

**Introduction**

There are three fundamental principles that I feel underpin the Ericksonian approach – Observation, Utilisation and having a Goal or Direction.

From these three fundamental principles much of the complexity of the Ericksonian approach develops naturally. When working with clients it is important to know what you are working towards or trying to achieve and to then make observations and utilise these observations in the direction of the goal. So, if a therapist observes that someone is anxious and holding on to the arm of the chair and the goal is to help them relax then they can utilise the gripping by suggesting "you can put all the tension in that grip" (focusing physical and emotional tension in one place), or "as you grip that arm of the chair with all of your tension I wonder how quickly you will relax" (presupposing relaxation and linking tension in the grip with relaxing). Or, "while you grip that arm of the chair another part of you can relax" (linking the gripping with relaxing), or "I don't know whether you will discover gripping the chair leads to relaxation spreading through the rest of your body, or whether you find your mind drifts and wanders and dreams" (linking gripping with a double bind – either the gripping with lead to relaxation, or the gripping will lead to the mind wandering and drifting into a dream-like state), or a whole range of other suggestions that are hypnotic language patterns, but the focus isn't on the language pattern, the language patterns develop naturally from utilising observations towards a goal.

**Observation**

Observation skills are something that therapists should continually practice and refine. When watching clients, observation is the key to discovering what to work with and feedback to the client. If a client twitches at a key point, perhaps in response to a specific idea being presented, or maybe at a point during a period of inner work, then the therapist would acknowledge this, all of the clients' micro-movements and unconscious movements can be acknowledged towards the desired goal. This goal may be the therapeutic goal, or it may be a series of goals, so firstly it could be the goal of developing trance, then the goal of going to a specific place in the mind, then to the goal of post hypnotic suggestions or future therapeutic success.

When I first learnt about congruency between conscious and unconscious messages I wanted to know how I could practice this and refine it as a skill. The best way I found was to watch people, watch them in bars, clubs, restaurants, parks, anywhere where you get to observe people interacting. By doing this you can listen to conversations at the same time as objectively watching non-verbal behaviour. Another place to watch this is on reality TV shows. I used to record reality TV shows each week and watch interactions between the people on the show to see what I could figure out about people based on mismatching communication. I would then make predictions based on my observations and watch future episodes of the show to see what predictions were accurate and which weren't and what I missed. As I got feedback from watching the shows I would refine and update my predictions. This is a great learning process.

You can watch people talking and look for patterns. Doing this you don't get to ask the questions but you can pay your full attention because you aren't involved. Anyone with knowledge of magic who watches a magician knows that if the magician is captivating enough people miss what they do even though they perhaps know what they were looking for and that sleight of hand or whatever it happened to be occurred right under their nose. This is the same when starting out doing therapy; you have lots of knowledge, you know what you can observe, but miss it when you are in a real situation because you have too much to take in and too much you are thinking about. As you watch people you may work by initially just getting a sense of something or you may actively look for patterns that you could tell someone else (like change in facial colour, change in the fullness of the lips, body posture, eye contact, etc.).

The best way to learn to recognise minimal cues is to focus on one cue at a time while you learn so that you get used to noticing that cue. Like focusing on observing the breathing pattern, or observing the pulse in the neck, or observing changes to skin colour or changes in the eyes. What you do with the observations depends on what you are observing for (it could be to look for congruence, or it could be for a specific state, etc.). If it is for a state then you can suggest back the minimal cues you observe for that state, so if you wanted to induce a deep trance comment or acknowledge the minimal cues (overtly or indirectly) each time you see a trance based minimal cue. You could link it to going deeper for example by saying "as you continue to blink in that special way you can drift deeper." Or "That's right" (said on each blink or sign of ideo-motor movement etc.). If you wanted to help the person develop a state of confidence then you would do this with minimal cues linked to that confidence like perhaps changes to voice tonality or straightening the back and putting the shoulders back. The easiest way of noticing minimal cues is to be in an externally focused trance on the client you are working with, this way you will be better able to notice and respond to minimal cues and see connections between the different cues you observe. This also develops with clinical practice and training, not just training around minimal cues, but also around what issues you are learning to treat.

To switch a client's trance focus (from internal to external or external to internal) you can start by matching the experience then guiding it to where it is wanted.

For example you could say to a client: "You can be aware of the ticking clock, of the traffic outside, of the sound of my breathing AND you can notice what those hands feel like resting on your lap WHILE you wonder what will happen next...and BEFORE you discover what will happen next you can notice which hand feels the heaviest and wonder whether one of those hands will lift... (Becoming more internally focused)"

To do this the other way reverse the process and match ongoing internal experience then you can ask the client to remain in this state while they open their eyes and pay their full attention honestly and completely to ... (whatever the external thing is - reading, practicing an instrument etc.)

With leisure activities you can have an external focus activity and guide it internally (even by saying "I sense you can feel some of that now").

Many people think too narrowly about observation. They perhaps look at breathing pattern, pulse, pupil dilation, head movements, changes to skin colour, blood flow to the lips, gestures, body position and movements and other physiological cues. Some people will also observe for language use, different emphasis the client gives to different words, what metaphors the client uses, their choice of words, any hesitations and other aspects auditory aspects of the ongoing situation. Building on this, some therapists may observe the wider situation, like sounds of traffic or other sounds in the building, any other distractions which occur, and any other environmental stimuli. This level of observation is just on what is occurring in the moment. What is needed is to broaden the observation out to include the client as a whole, things like: what type of person are they? What is their family history? What is/was their place in the family? What does this inform you about how they may respond to things? What types of jobs have they done? How do they respond to different types of situations? What is important to them? What do they enjoy? What motivates them/makes them passionate to take action, etc? What is their wider life like? What meets their different innate needs? What are their hopes and dreams? What do they want life to be like now/in the future, etc?

You also want to broaden your observations to include your learnings, so for example, if a client says they are depressed and you know about the cycle of depression I would class this knowledge as an observation to be utilised. Just knowing the cycle of depression means when a client tells you that they are depressed, you can talk about sleep difficulties you know they are likely to have, you can talk about worry thinking they are likely to do, you can talk about them feeling exhausted and struggling with motivation. It maybe that for the specific client they don't have all these issues, but your knowledge gives you a starting point, something that can likely be utilised. You will also know that the client is likely to have one or more innate needs not being met, or being inappropriately met, so you know to explore this, so you are utilising your knowledge, or, in this case, your observations about what it means for someone to be depressed.

The more the therapist learns about different things, from child developmental psychology, social psychology, whatever issues you will be working with and any issues which may arise with clients in therapy as well as about different cultural and religious viewpoints, the better able to draw on this information the therapist will be, and the more they will have access to utilise when working with the client. Learning the three principles of the Ericksonian approach is easy, but to master applying the Ericksonian approach takes learning and extensive practice. Effective therapists will continue to practice and study and develop themselves. If they have a client with an interest that they don't know much about they will learn something about that interest so that they can better help the client.

When I worked in children's homes, whenever a new child was coming into the home we would receive the child's care plan a few days beforehand. This care plan would say many things about the child including their hobbies and interests and things like their favourite football team. I have no interest in football, but I would always go and learn a bit about the subjects in the care plan so that I could interact meaningfully with the child when they come into the home. I would learn about their favourite football team and how well (or badly) they are currently doing, how they have done over recent years, any significant changes over recent years, any planned changes in the near future, any significant games which have been played and which are to be played, what kits they wear, where they are located in the country. I've got no idea about football, but I want to be able to be authentic in my interactions and it could arise that I have something helpful to say, or something I need to address with them and being able to use their interest and communicate from within something they know, love and understand is very helpful. This is the kind of thing I expect of good therapists. It is all much easier now with the internet. When I was doing this, I used to have to go to a library to find all the information out.

The best way to observe successfully is to observe with curiosity, so you watch people and wonder about what you observe. If you see a possible pattern, wonder "What was that about? Why did they do that?"

Watch clients and look for patterns. Anyone that has knowledge of magic and watches a magician knows that if the magician is captivating enough you miss what they do even though you know it happened right under your nose. This is the same when starting out doing therapy; you know lots of stuff but miss it when you are in a real situation because you have too much to take in. Practice by watching people. As you watch people you may work by initially just getting a sense of something or you may actively look for patterns that you could tell someone else (like change in facial colour, change in lips, body posture, eye contact, etc.). Often therapists focus on the content of problems. It is more helpful to focus on the pattern of the problem. For the problem to be a problem there will be a pattern playing out. This pattern may happen across contexts, so many seemingly unrelated issues may actually be related. You may not discover what initially caused the original pattern, but you can find the one pattern that is happening in many areas and address that one pattern. When observing the therapist can look for patterns in behaviour that reveal additional information, like someone rubbing their neck while talking about a partner and when the therapist changes the subject and returns to talking about their partner they do the same again implying the person is a *pain in the neck,* or while they tell you they want to change you see them pushing their feet into the ground, and again when the therapist changes the subject and then returns to it they do the same again communicating that they are *digging their heels in* about the issue of changing and perhaps are unlikely to be ready to change yet.

It is important to check out observations. Many years ago, I was in a job interview and kept putting my right arm across my lap and my left arm over my right arm holding it in place. I had just recently been hit by a truck and sustained significant injuries to my right arm so, whenever I sat on a chair without suitable armrests I would rest my arm across my lap and hold it in place with my other arm as this was the most comfortable position and gave me the least pain.

Following the interview I got to see the interviewers' notes, the interviewers were trained in neuro-linguistic programming (NLP) and so had learned about observation skills, however what they wrote about the interview was that most of the time I had my arms crossed on my lap and so was clearly defensive and resistant and reluctant to be open and honest. They clearly hadn't checked out their observations and remained open-minded until the evidence pointed in a specific direction. They didn't check whether I was crossing my arms because I was cold, or whether, as was the case, I was crossing my arms for comfort due to an injury. I had been open and honest in telling them about recently being involved in a road accident, being hospitalised and sustaining significant injuries to my arm, but they didn't link this information I had told them to my ongoing behaviour, they didn't ask questions then change topics and come back to the topic and see if I repeated the behaviour, or just ask me something like "I'm curious about you crossing your arms?"

To check out your observations, you can change the topic or do something else to change the state of the client, and then return to the topic again and see if the client goes to doing the same behaviour once you change back to the topic. You can also ask them about behaviours and observations and observe how they respond.

Here is a selection of minimal cues that can be observed, it is helpful to make observations for utilisation and for deeper understanding. For example, if there is a mismatch between the conscious and non-conscious communication. This can be utilised, but also it teaches a lot about the person and their presenting problem or solution. Generally, if there is a mismatch in communication, the non-conscious communication is likely to be the honest, authentic communication, but to know this for sure the therapist needs to test their observations:

- Heartbeat – looking in the ankle, temple, throat
- Facial colour changes – reddening, whitening of the face
- Eye movements
- Eye contact
- Tension and relaxation in parts of the face or other parts of the body

- Thickening or narrowing of lips – due to blood flow
- Tensing or relaxing of lips
- Head position
- Head movement
- Eyes widening or narrowing
- Micro-expressions
- Throat movements
- Swallowing
- Body position
- Body posture
- Arm, hand, feet or leg movements
- Position of arms, hands, feet, or legs
- Differences and similarities between verbal reports and non-verbal behaviour
- Metaphorical behaviours
- Tone of voice
- Speed of speech
- Pauses and emphasis given during speech

- Quality of speech
- Types of words used
- Amount of information, or type of information given or not spoken
- Subtle changes to speech, like wavering voice, change in pitch or firmer voice
- Gestures used
- Breathing rate and type of breathing, and changes to breathing – like hesitant breathing or holding breath at certain times or breathing faster or slower depending on what is going on at the time
- Perspiration
- Metaphors used
- Patterns
- Self-soothing/self-punishing behaviours
- Anxiety behaviours

## Utilisation

There are so many observations which can be utilised. What you decide to utilise and how will depend on the individual client and on what the goal is. The aim utilisation is to find a client-centred way of achieving the goal rather than trying to make the client fit the therapists' way that the goal should be achieved. A therapist using an Ericksonian approach would always be focusing on what observations they have and how these can be utilised towards the goal the client wants to achieve. If the client starts to tell the therapist about the weather and how nice it is outside, they can use this to elicit pleasant feelings or to encourage them to think about a holiday that can be used to relax them or utilised in some other way.

To utilise feelings that the client mentions, it is important to feedback what they say in a way that gets them more absorbed into those feelings in the present (if that is the aim). For example, if a client was talking about a time they felt good about an achievement, as you talk to them you can begin to re-evoke those feelings in the present and begin to associate them with solving the problem. To do this you need to feedback what they say into present tense. So, the client may have said "I completed a 10-kilometre run a few years back. I didn't think I could do it and was so pleased when I crossed the finish line." The therapist could reply asking questions about how it felt, how they knew they felt pleased, asking them to think back and absorb themselves in the memory. They can ask "where did the good feeling of achievement start in your body?" Then when the client replies stating something like "it started in my stomach." The therapist can follow this up with something like "it starts in your stomach." Then they can pause a moment for the feeling in the present to develop further before asking something like "and what happens next with that feeling?" This begins to have the client focusing on the feeling in the present, rather than just the memory. The therapist could then use anchoring to link the elicited feeling with a tone of voice or a touch so that it can be triggered later when the client is thinking of something where that feeling would be helpful.

The therapist can use all sorts of emotions and responses whether it is anger or resistance or lack of motivation or positive things like having a supportive family, being confident at playing a musical instrument, running a marathon each year, or a pleasant experience, whatever it happens to be. A therapist can channel a client's anger towards being angry at an addiction bullying them, or their resistance to do therapeutic tasks into resistance to doing the problem behaviours, or lack of motivation to having a lack of motivation doing problem behaviour, or having a supportive family could be used to help them develop a support network to keep them on track with the therapy, confidence playing a musical instrument could have the confidence transferred to being confident public speaking, if the problem was licking confidence public speaking. The tenacity and ability not to give up and to run a marathon, which means they also have the motivation to do hard work of training for a marathon and are able to do something which at times will be unpleasant and push through and keep going because they know they want the end result, this can be channelled to help the client keep going, working hard and working towards achieving their goals. Most things that the therapist observes can be used to help the client. They will be communicating their way that things need to be done. So, a client with a problem they can't seem to overcome, but who runs marathons has the skills; there is something about the running marathons situation which allows these skills to be present, it is just a question now of how this can be transferred so that whatever it is they do to be motivated to run marathons can happen in relation to achieving their therapeutic goals.

An example of utilising the feelings from what a client has said:

Client: "I went out for a walk in the country the other day. It was so relaxing."

Therapist: "What was it you find so relaxing?" (Intentionally using "find" instead of "found")

Client: "All the different colours, the cool breeze, the feeling of the warm sun on my face." (The client has to become more absorbed – deepen their trance – in the experience to give more detail)

Therapist: "So, you see all the different colours, feel that cool breeze and the warm sun on your face." (Encouraging the client to become deeper absorbed in the experience they are sharing, but in the present rather than the past)

Client: "Yes." (Getting agreement because all I am saying is what I have been told. The agreement encourages further future agreement and has the client agreeing with going deeper into the experience they are having here and now)

You can anchor to link a resource with solving their problem, or you can encourage them to rehearse hypnotically utilising resources. Rehearsing hypnotically doesn't mean putting the client into a formal hypnotic trance, it means creating an experience in the mind of the client that is focused on what is helpful for them to focus on. With practice utilisation becomes easier, and resources begin to stand out as if they are marked with neon markers.

Almost everything the client says and does is right for helping to treat them. When I am doing therapy I constantly use what the client says and does to get them to where they want to go. I regularly tell them "that's right" or "mmm" or do something that is acknowledging to them that they are doing the right thing to go into a trance or to quit smoking or whatever it happens to be.

For example, if someone comes to me for therapy and says "I'm too stressed to be able to relax and go into hypnosis." I'll tell them "That's excellent. All the best work is done with the clients that have some tension there. What I need you to do is just hold on to some of that tension for a while as we do this."

If a client says "You won't be able to hypnotise me because I'm too strong willed." I'll tell them "You're right I won't be able to hypnotise you, all I can do is guide you into a state of mind that gives you greater control over the inner workings of your mind and body. A state of mind that allows you to control your heart rate, your blood pressure, your breathing and many other processes, but it takes a strong-willed person to enter that state fully and completely."

One quick way to induce a trance is to have a person recall their problem (it is often likely to be trance inducing), like getting a smoker to recall smoking (or getting a craving), or a person in pain to focus on the pain (only this time in a non-attached way, focusing on its colour, shape, size, etc.), or a person that has OCD to discuss their OCD process, or someone with a spider phobia to recall the phobia, etc. The higher the level of emotion the deeper the trance the person will naturally go into when they recall it. You're always working with the trances you get; some people are just more responsive than others and so would appear to be better hypnotic subjects. Everybody is different; some people you can just look at them and say sleep and they will (if they know you do hypnosis and expect it to happen) go into a *hypnotic sleep*. Others would not respond in this way. A good hypnotic subject is likely to be able to perform a wide variety of hypnotic phenomena, but just because someone perhaps can't hallucinate, or doesn't visualise clearly in their mind, or whatever it may be, doesn't mean they won't respond well to therapy.

As Milton Erickson used to mention, in some cases he had to train people for some time to help them to be good hypnotic subjects (Erickson M. H., 1952). When you are hypnotising someone, you are looking for responsivity to what you say. If they happen to be great at any specific hypnotic phenomena then these can be utilised in the therapy.

Something to consider is that it can be helpful to notice when people enter naturally, drift deeper into trance. It could be for example, that the therapist has just offered an interpretation of a situation that the client hadn't thought about before and so they stare off into space while they consider and process what has been said and are updating their neurology with this new information. When the therapist notices this they would want to give the client some time to finish this inner work. They wouldn't want to keep talking and asking questions and interrupting the client's natural flow. If they do talk to the client, they would want to lower their voice and be as unobtrusive as possible.

When utilising the problem itself all the therapist has to do is ask about the stages of the problem the client has and their trance will deepen around the pattern of the problem for them to access the information to tell the therapist. If the therapist asks the client about a leisure activity they enjoy, they will deepen their trance to go inside their mind to access this information, if they are then asked for more detail they have to become even more absorbed in the experience to access this information. If the therapist asks a client what colour their front door is, the client will deepen their trance and asking for more details, again, will deepen that trance further. Asking a client how they will know when they are better will again, may lead to the client going deeper into a trance narrowing their focus on this information. These are all small and simple ways of initiating a focusing of attention just by utilising aspects of everyday human experience and responsivity.

You can utilise past hypnosis experiences. It is helpful to find out if the client has had any prior experience with hypnosis, to find out what that was, whether it worked for them, what their thoughts are about that prior experience, how they were hypnotised, etc. If a therapist asks a client "have you ever been in a hypnotised before?" what they are doing is a double bind. This is because they have added the word *before*. If they ask "have you ever been hypnotised?", the client can answer "yes" or "no", if they add the word *before* it means before something, but before what? Before being hypnotised now? Before being hypnotised shortly? So, whether they answer yes or no they are accepting they will either go into hypnosis or are already hypnotised.

If they answer "yes" and it was a positive or therapeutic experience then gathering information about that prior hypnotic trance experience will quickly guide them back into a similar trance again yet it will appear like the therapist was just enquiring about that previous trance. If the therapist wants to still follow this line of questioning to induce hypnosis when the client has said that they haven't been hypnotised before they can just explain what it will be like to be hypnotised (using your hypnotic language skills) and start utilising the client's ongoing experience by describing this as part of what the experience of being hypnotised is like which will guide the client into hypnosis. Either way they are likely to enter a hypnotic state rapidly and be well on their way before they know what is happening.

To work with an Ericksonian approach the therapist needs to let go of scripts and focus on being client-centred. It doesn't mean that between sessions the therapist doesn't write down ideas of things which could be helpful to cover with the client, like perhaps writing down some of the client's metaphors and writing down ideas for how these could be used, but they don't write down or use scripts directly with the client where they would be staring at a script and using the script rather than focusing on the client during the session.

I just wanted to share my experiences of stopping using scripts and moving on to hypnosis using observation, utilisation and a goal. When I first trained, all of my training was direct and all about using scripts. Courses would teach a handful of inductions which you would read to clients, they would give you a handful of therapeutic scripts to read to clients or recommend some books you can find scripts in to read to clients. There was no therapeutic knowledge taught in these courses. The expectation was that you would learn the scripts, then read an induction to the client followed by direct suggestions telling the client they will no longer have their problem and then tell them to exit hypnosis. I contacted every therapist in my area to learn from them, get their opinions and views on their success etc. and all the feedback was to buy lots of scripts and when a client tells you what their problem is, use a script for that, find out which induction script they want and use that and use a script for ending the therapy. I had a collection of over 500 scripts! Imagine sitting with a client and trying to remember which script I should use! I also felt it was wrong to just read in a monotonous voice from a sheet of paper and get paid for it and claim I knew what I was doing. They could buy a book of scripts, choose the ones that suited them best and audio record the script themselves for much cheaper than paying for therapy.

When I found out about Ericksonian Hypnosis, I realised what I should be doing, and it wasn't just memorising and reciting inductions and therapy scripts demanding clients will be problem free, it was tailoring the therapy and hypnosis to the client. I attended a two-day course on Ericksonian Hypnosis with Uncommon Knowledge in Brighton, UK. On the course we had to sit opposite someone and (like the TV quiz show catchphrase) 'say what you see'. This was fine and I was comfortable with this in the safety of a course where at least I knew I could do hypnosis and was already confident doing hypnosis, there were beginners that had never done hypnosis before. By this point I had also started 'ad-libbing' self-help tracks because I couldn't find tracks or scripts for what I wanted to explore and had been doing hypnosis for about ten years but hadn't yet fully let go of my script crutches. I had learned about hypnotic language patterns and tonality and had been studying the work of Milton H Erickson, but I still used scripts with client because I thought I would not know what to say if I didn't have a *professional script* in front of me.

After the course I met up with a friend that was willing to be a guinea pig, I said confidently that I can now do hypnosis without using scripts (having only done this on the training course, and from some of my personal self-hypnosis tapes and CD's). I decided I would do a leisure induction with him and utilise his interests and times his mind has naturally wandered and utilise on-going behaviours that I observe in him. I asked him "in an ideal world where you could do anything, what would you do that would make your mind wander, that would make you lose track of time and really enjoy yourself?"

His response was "I would go back to Thunder Mountain" (apparently some water-ride in America?).

I thought to myself 'well I said I would use anything', so I did and he said it was the deepest trance he had ever been in and we got numerous hypnotic phenomenon and great success. I was nervous when he didn't say a nice warm beach or something like all the course participants had said, but I am glad that he didn't because it helped with my learning, development and confidence as a hypnotherapist and I have never looked back and now can't imagine using scripts with clients. The thing I learned was that you can't be wrong because you are given your script moment by moment by paying attention. If you expect the client to be hypnotised and so let your voice and breathing guide them it doesn't matter if you don't yet know all of the language patterns. You learn best by being uncertain at first rather than knowing it all then deciding to try it out.

## An example of me utilising describing my own experience to induce hypnosis

"You know one of my interests is going on walks through the nearby woods. I'll spend hours just *wandering* along in my own world...*feeling the breeze on your skin*...I...begin to *notice the sound of each footstep*...time seems to just... *slow right down*...and I seem to be able to ...*notice the smoothness of the movement of breathing*, of each regular step, of individual sounds from the birds, the rustling of the leaves...*noticing the shimmering rays of light*...the warmth of the sun on my face...and as I continue walking I...*notice how the breathing begins to relax and deepen all by itself*...often I find my...*muscles relaxing*...around my shoulders, arms, neck and face...and before long it already seems like time to go home..."

When a therapist talks hypnotically about an interest the client often finds it a familiar experience and so gets guided indirectly by listening to the description. I did this for one person (a hypnotherapist) where I challenged myself to see if I could hypnotise a hypnotist without them noticing I was hypnotising them. Part of what I did was said "you know I've always wanted to drive down America, *see how things change on a journey through the States* *and* I went into detail about this imaginary journey in conversation and he was hypnotised in no time at all and didn't notice it happening, he just became increasingly responsive and started to drift into his mind.

I often tell hypnotherapists that they should start everything with agreement and then figure out how to move on from there. So, if the therapist doesn't get the response they are after, that is fine, the response they are getting is the correct one for this moment in time. This goes for therapy as well as when inducing hypnosis. I had a client who asked if her husband could sit in the session because she had never been hypnotised before and was scared about it. I was working with her to help her quit smoking. At the end of the session the husband said that he was surprised at how natural his wife seemed to be at all this, because she did everything right and got all the responses expected of her. I agreed that she responded to everything and was thinking about how she had barely responded as I had hoped to anything, but this was okay, she responded as was right for her from moment to moment. If I tried to get an arm levitation and the arm just sat there not moving I utilised this and said "or will that arm be so heavy it just rests there on your lap?" So, whatever happened I used as being the correct thing to be happening in that moment and linked it with the desired goals.

**Goal**

*"If a client doesn't give the response that you expect then utilise what they do give you and acknowledge that what they are doing is what they need to do to achieve the desired goal."*

Without setting goals you would have no idea of knowing when you have reached the time to end therapy. Without setting goals you also don't know exactly what the client needs or what to say to them about what they hope to gain from the therapy. The ultimate goal of therapy for the therapist is to try to get clients to a point where you never have to see them again, as quickly as possible.

Goal setting is a vital part of the process of effective therapy. You need to ask questions that establish what the client wants to achieve and how they expect it to impact on their life in the future. You need to use high quality information gathering to build up a picture of the goals that are required. These goals can then be used to focus your mind on what you need to do to help the client get what it is that they want from therapy. You have immediate goals of what the client would like to get during the session and from this session, at least one overall goal is the answer to "How will you know when you no longer have to see me again? What will life be like for you?" And within this there will be intermediate goals that are things which are the steps between where the client is at and where they want to be. Sometimes there are things which need to happen before the client is likely to be able to create the lasting change they want. For example, a smoker may need to learn relaxation skills, or how to be assertive, or some other skills or address some other issues, before being able to quit smoking for good. Goals need to be SMART – Specific, Measurable, Achievable, Realistic and Time-bound. They also need to be fully under the control of the client. So, it isn't a SMART goal saying "I want my child to behave.", because this is stating someone else's actions that they want to be different and only that other person can decide to alter their actions. A SMART goal may be "I want to be able to remain calm and keep to a clear message when my son isn't doing as I have asked." The therapist can ask a scaling question like "on a scale of 0-10, with 10 being that you are behaving in that way with your son all the time and 0 being the opposite, where are you now?" This type of question and related follow up questions will make it measurable. The therapist will be looking for visual, auditory and kinaesthetic answers from the client, often described as *video-speak*, so what would they observe if they were following the client around with a camcorder. If the client for example rated that currently they are at a 2 out of 10, then the therapist would establish what makes them say 2 and not 1, what is it they are seeing, hearing, doing, feeling that makes it 2 not 1. They would ask what would make it 3, so they now get from the client a video-speak description for 3. They can ask the client what number they would be happy with, given nothing is perfect. So, 10 is that they are always doing the desired way of handling their child. Often people will say 7 or 8. If they say 8, then the therapist can ask the client what an 8 would be like, how would they know they are at an 8? They can be asked "at what point would you feel you probably don't need my help and can probably continue to make progress from this point on your own?" This is an important question, because often beyond a certain point the client doesn't need the therapists help, for example, if someone wanted to lose weight there would be a point where all they are doing in sessions is reporting their weight loss, there is nothing new for the therapist to help them with other than monitoring progress until the goal and the client may not need this. In the parenting example, the parent may have things pretty much under control and things could be generally going well with just a few blips, but they may be confident that they have the skills and knowledge now not to need to pay to see a therapist because all they need to do is continue to practice and keep doing what they are doing and they will reach that 8 out of 10 which they would be happy with. It could be that a 6 or 7 would be the point they no longer need to see a therapist. They may say at this point they would be happy just knowing they can see the therapist if needed, or if they can book an appointment for a month or two in the future to see that they are still on track and doing okay.

Once the therapist has the SMART goal that is about what the client will be changing and doing differently, then observations made can be utilised towards this goal and aspects of the goal or any of the stages which have been observed can be utilised. For example, if a parent said "just having one meal together as a family a week would move me from a 2 to a 3." Then the therapist can start working on what it would take for the family to sit down and have a meal together and at some point would set a task for the parent to commit to a day when that family meal will happen and have the family meal. As soon as the family has that meal this means the parent's rating will have moved from 2 to 3. This is a big step, sometimes there are small details which are easy to achieve that people describe as part of their description for a number on the scale. When something can easily be done these work really well to be utilised and set as tasks and when the client then starts doing these things that means they are already closer to the goal and will start rating where they are at higher.

As long as the goal is SMART then there is no reason why it wouldn't be achievable meaning that the therapist can take an attitude of expecting that the goal will be achieved, the only questions are how and when. I find this is one of the most liberating and helpful attitudes to have. As soon as I approached hypnosis as something inevitable for clients, it was just a question of how and when for them, hypnosis became easy, all of my questions were about observing the client and because of the expectation that they will become hypnotised (as the goal) I was just utilising whatever observations I had as curiosity about how and when. I think this is one of the most important attitudes to develop. If what you are told is something you have no doubt that the client can achieve or experience, then just be curious and focus on how and when they will achieve that, not if they might. This goes for hypnosis and therapy. If you can do this then your therapeutic practice and ease with which you approach clients and your client-centred approach will significantly improve. You will use all of the hypnotic language patterns and various technique naturally whether you know them or not because they all come from curiosity and expectancy and just exploring how and when the client will be successful.

## Pacing and leading

The idea behind nearly all hypnotic techniques is pacing and leading, you want to pace your observations of where someone currently is and then lead them to somewhere else. It can go from any point to any other point. The best linguistic techniques for this are compound suggestions and contingent suggestions and presuppositions. The first two use linking terms like 'and, before, during, after, while, as' these naturally pace and lead. The leap you make will depend on the individual and how big the gap is between where they are and where they want to be. For example, in therapy it could be:

"You've come here today to see me (pacing) because you want to see how I can help (leading but still likely to be true so not a huge leap, and presupposing I can help)"

"And you don't yet know how I'm going to be able to help you (pacing and presupposition) but you're probably curious to find out (leading)"

"Before I explain how I can help (presupposition that I will help) I wonder if you can tell me what you would like (linking being told with getting help)"

In everyday situations:

"As you go into the kitchen (pacing) could you flick the kettle on (leading)"

"You appear to want to continue shouting and ignoring me (pacing) and don't yet want to listen (leading - yet implies/presupposes in the future you will want to listen)"

To build rapport and good relationships you have to begin by pacing another person. Pacing is when you enter the other person's model of the world. It is like walking beside them at their speed. Too fast and they will have to hurry to keep up with you, too slow and they have to hold themselves back. Either way they have to make a special effort. The therapist is the one that should be making the special effort for the benefit of making the client relaxed and comfortable with them.

Once you have paced another person, and gained rapport and shown that you understand where they're coming from, then you can lead them. To pace the client, you can either do matching, cross-matching or mirroring depending on the situation and which feels right for the circumstances. Trust your feelings, they will usually be right.

Matching is where the therapist does the same as the client, so if the client moves their right arm, so does the therapist. Cross-matching is where the therapist matches the client with something different, so the client moves their right arm, and the therapist moves their left leg. Or the client is tapping their foot, so the therapist taps a finger, or the therapist is watching the client's pulse and matches this with a foot movement. Mirroring is where the therapist is like a mirror of the client, so if they move their right arm, the therapist moves their left arm the same. The idea isn't to mimic the client, but to be similar to the client. There is nothing more annoying than someone copying everything you are doing. The idea is to be like the person, so if they use a specific type of gesture when they say something, or make a specific movement, then if you say similar or are thinking about similar things then you do similar. So, if the therapist asks a probing question and then the client sits back in their chair to think about what they have been asked, when a similar situation happens for the therapist where they think deeply about a question they have been asked, they would then sit back in their chair in a similar way as they think about the answer. So, it isn't about mimicking, it is about being similar to the client so that they feel like you share their way of processing the world.

# Priming

Priming is presenting ideas to stimulate patterns. Milton Erickson used to call this seeding. He would talk about seeding ideas to allow the idea to develop before needing it (Zeig, 1980). We have covered priming significantly already in the first *Hypnotherapy Revealed* volume: *Introduction to Hypnotherapy*, but it is covered here a little more because it specifically comes into something that Erickson used to do a lot of as part of the Ericksonian approach. An example of priming would be if a therapist wanted to get an arm levitation they could present ideas about levitation, lifting arms, and automatic movement, and then when they actually go to elicit the arm levitation the neural patterns for levitation will already be active. It could be that they talk about things like a child feeling the overwhelming urge to want to get teachers attention when they know the answer to a question in class or trying to get something down from the top shelf in the kitchen cupboard. If the therapist would like the client to think about their relationship with their father then they could talk about relationships and childhood and their own father, all of which would make the client think about their father.

Priming is like booting up computer software in the background so that when you need it the software opens once you click on it, rather than not booting it up in advance and then turning it on when you need it and then having to wait for ages for it to load before you can use it. In priming research people presented with stereotypes take on their understanding of some of the traits associated with those stereotypes. When people see things associated with the stereotype for glamour models, they do worse on IQ tests, when people see things associated with the stereotype for scientists, they do better on IQ tests. When people see things associated with the stereotype for children they increase in apparent fitness and reaction times and can walk faster for example, and when people see things associated with the stereotype for elderly they decrease in fitness and reaction times and walk slower for example.

When people hold a warm drink the pattern for warmth is stimulated, meaning if they are then asked how much they like someone they generally answer more favourably due to feeling that they *warm* to the person. When people hold a cold drink the pattern for cold is stimulated, meaning if they are then asked how much they like someone they generally answer less favourably due to feeling *cold* towards that person. We talk about warm-hearted, warmed to them, cold-hearted, they appeared really cold.

These metaphors are part of our language and can be primed through language and physically. Priming is complex. Take cold for example, being presented with a cold drink may prime for coldness and if that person is then asked to rate how friendly someone is while they are primed with coldness they may rate them lower. If it is a really hot day and someone is given a cold drink to hold they may feel pleasure in holding that cold drink which may prevent the coldness prime working.

Likewise, if they are snuggled up in a tent with a loved one when it is cold outside and they are a little chilly in the tent, you would think they are primed with coldness, but there is a lot of other things going on which probably have more influence, like the meaning behind the experience and perhaps they also feel love towards the other person in the situation as they share the experience.

# Hypnotic Language Patterns: The Agreement Set

**Pattern of agreement**

The agreement set is probably the most basic class of hypnotic language pattern. The aim of it is to get agreement with the client. The therapist is aiming for a pattern of agreement that begins to be habitual agreement so that the client becomes more likely to continue to agree.

For example:

Therapist: "So, your name is Dan"

Client: "Yes"

Therapist: "And you live at... (stating the client's address)"

Client: "Yes"

Therapist: "And you booked the appointment about a week ago"

Client: "Yes"

Therapist: "And you said you wanted help with anxiety"

Client: "Yes"

Therapist: "And you're not seeing a doctor currently about that anxiety (assuming you know the answer is no)"

Client: "No"

Therapist: "Thank you, so let's see what we can do about the anxiety. You're sat in that chair, listening to me speak, probably curious about what I am going to say"

Client: "Yes"

What each of these statements has in common is that they get agreement from the client. I have written them here with responses, but it could just as easily be implied agreement responses, so the therapist could be *talking to themselves* about the facts on the referral form and not to the client. So, they ask the client to take a seat and then they get the referral form out and start reading through it to themselves, not directly to the client, just saying to themselves "so your name is Dan, you live at..., you booked the session a week ago and said that you want help with anxiety." The therapist may not look up from the page the whole time they say this. The client may not verbalise answers but will still be agreeing with them in their mind, and still building up a pattern of agreement. Once this pattern of agreement has formed the therapist can offer leading suggestions and these are more likely to be accepted by the client.

## Truisms

Truisms are at the heart of many of these hypnotic language patterns. A truism is a statement of fact, it is undeniable. If a client is sitting in a chair and the therapist says "you are sitting in that chair." Then this would be true, and so would be a truism. If the therapist says "you are wondering what I am thinking." This isn't a truism unless the therapist knows this for sure somehow. It may be true, but if the therapist doesn't know it to be true then it may also be false. Generally, most of what a therapist says they want to say because they already know it to be true. These would often also be pacing statements. If the therapist is going to say something which may not be true, it is best to have gained a pattern of agreement first and then initially introducing things which could be true. So, it could be true that the client is wondering what the therapist is thinking. It is less likely to be true that they see a dog sat at their feet (when you know there is no dog at their feet). Yet, later in a session when perhaps the therapist has elicited some smaller level hallucinations, the client would be more likely to accept a suggestion that a dog is sat by their feet.

In my example above, I ended with a leading suggestion which may not be true. They may not be curious about what I am going to say. Because I will have gained a pattern of agreement by the time I suggest that, there is an increased chance of it being correct. Because I say "probably" I am not saying they definitely will be thinking that, so if they aren't it shouldn't impact on the flow of the session too much, but the likelihood is that they will just follow it, even if they actually weren't curious until I suggested that they might be.

**Yes set**

The *yes set* can help with verbal pacing and leading. If you get the client to say or think "yes" a number of times they become more likely to continue to respond with a "yes" response and because the conversation is all agreeable they feel more understood which paces them and makes them easier to lead. There are many children's games like this, like Simon Says (the game where you have to do what Simon says, but not do what is said if the person giving the suggestions didn't say "Simon says" before the suggestion), where you say something over and over again "Simon says... Simon says... Simon says... Simon says..." and then you get told "sit down." Without "Simon says" and many people will automatically sit down and most of those who don't sit down will hesitate a moment and will have felt the urge to follow the suggestion because they were in a pattern of following what was being said.

The best way to guarantee a 'yes' and improve rapport is to ask what you know to be true as you continue to gain rapport then lead with an attached statement or suggestion.

For example:

- "You are sitting in that chair"
- "You've come here today to see me"

These statements can only lead to a yes answer if they are true which means that you are increasing rapport, because rapport increases with agreement and understanding. It also builds up a response potential. It gets harder to disagree when you have been repeatedly in agreement.

Don't make all the answers verbal "yes" answers some of the answers elicited should be implied yes answers.

For example:

- "You look like someone who wants to get better?"

It is increasingly hard to disagree when you have been agreeing to many questions. One easy way of getting agreement is to feedback what the client says. It sounds like you are clarifying but you are getting agreement.

For example:

Client: "I don't know what's wrong with me."

Therapist: "You don't know what's wrong with you..."

Client: "No." (It is a *no* answer, but this no means "I agree")

**Reverse yes set**

The reverse yes set is the same as above but always getting "no" answers. By using a mixture of the reverse yes set, the yes set and implied agreement, you can break up the questions. If you ask too many questions where the person is just saying "yes" or just saying "no" every answer, this doesn't flow or seem natural and can feel to the client like the therapist is trying to manipulate them.

The answers are still all agreement

- "So, you're not standing up"
- "And you didn't drive here this morning"
- "And you wouldn't expect to go into hypnosis before you were ready"

All said assuming the therapist knows the answers to these questions already so that they are true statements (truisms).

*If the client shakes their head when you want agreement start shaking your head subtly also to create behavioural rapport then merge it into a nod.*

# HYPNOTIC LANGUAGE PATTERNS: LINKING SUGGESTIONS

**Direction**

Linking suggestions are suggestions that build on each other. They link things together that may not always be connected in reality; making it seem like because one thing has happened or is true the next thing should also then happen or be true. Linking suggestions build on the agreement set and like the agreement set, they are best done using truisms as the core of what you are doing.

The two main types of linking suggestions are compound suggestions and contingent suggestions. With compound suggestions, often the linking is done with an "and" or with a pause and the first part is usually a truism *pacing* statement whilst the second part doesn't necessarily have to be true but it leads on from the previous statement. To start with it is often best to use pacing and leading truisms. Sometimes this can just come down to wording. If a therapist says "you will relax", this might not be true. If they say "you can relax", this is true, everyone can relax.

Whereas with contingent suggestions often the linking is done with time-based words like "before, during, after, as, while". Again, they often start with truisms and then lead the client in a specific direction (pacing and leading). Another pattern that can be used is "don't...until" which works well for people that are more likely to be resistant because you as the therapist then state the negative before the client does, often preventing them from saying it. For example, if a client was doing the opposite of what the therapist was suggesting, or they had a "yes, but" attitude where they challenged everything and felt nothing would work, then if the therapist says "don't go into hypnosis until you are ready." The implication is that they will go into hypnosis and that this will happen when they are ready, but that there is a chance of them going into hypnosis before they are ready so they are being told not to do this but to wait until they are ready. Most clients who are polarity responders, people who do the opposite of what they are told, will often then go into hypnosis quicker because they were told not to until they were ready. Those who respond negatively to everything, who may say they can't be hypnotised often accept this suggestion. The client says they can't be hypnotised and the therapist replies with "that's okay, don't go into hypnosis until you are ready", changes it from the client having their black-and-white viewpoint of not being able to be hypnotised, to, they won't be hypnotised until they are ready. This now just makes it a matter of time, not whether it is possible or not.

## Compound suggestions

Compound suggestions are suggestions where you are pacing and then leading suggestions onto each other, building on the previous sentence (pacing is where you match the client's model of reality and state what you know to be true for the client; leading is where you add on something extra for the client to follow even if it doesn't really connect with what is paced). This is usually done by starting with pacing observable truisms then leading towards the response you want. The idea is to give a statement followed by a suggestion as if they are really linked together. By giving sentences linked to previous sentences you are compounding one suggestion onto the next and so deepening the effects.

One part compounds onto the next. Link these suggestions with 'and' or a 'pause'

For example:

- "Look at that spot and I will talk to you." (Pace and then lead)
- "While you look at that spot (pacing), I will talk to you (leading)."

Use truisms or statements then lead with a suggestion or further truisms or statements

For example:

- "You can listen to my voice (pacing and linked to previous sentence in the last example), and you can hear other sounds (leading)."
- "Some sounds evoke pleasant memories (pacing, linked to the previous sentence and a truism) and you can be interested to discover what images are associated with those memories (leading)."

Use a number of suggestions together one after the other linking them all to guide a client from where they are to where they want to be.

For example:

- "You can look at that spot (pacing) while I talk to you (leading)."

- "While I talk to you, you can listen (pacing) and you can begin to get a sense of how you will know when things start to improve in the future (leading)."

- "And I don't know which improvements will happen first (pacing) and you can relax a little deeper as those improvements come to mind (leading)."

Example compound suggestions:

- "You can look at me and begin to relax."

- "You can relax and think of pleasant memories."

- "You can be thinking of those pleasant memories and wonder what you can learn from them."

As you may have noticed above you can also use compound suggestions to guide people from external reality to internal reality. So above I started with what I could see (they are looking at me) which also means they are focusing externally. Then I mentioned they can relax which begins to focus them internally. Then thinking of pleasant memories which focuses them deeper on an internal reality and less on external reality. Then finally had them wonder what they can learn from this which increases the focus on having to now find something to learn.

Compound suggestions can overlap. Generally, it is a truism followed by a suggestion; this can be from observable to non-observable, out of trance to in trance, etc.

For example:

- "You can sit there and read this writing."
- "You can read this writing and let thoughts come to mind."
- "Those thoughts can come to mind and some can be of pleasant experiences."
- "You can be aware of those pleasant experiences and become more absorbed and relaxed."

One thing I did when initially learning this and all of the other language patterns and structures was to listen to conversations (in real life and on TV) and look out for specific patterns.

In work, lots of times people would say things like "Your shift doesn't finish for another hour, does it? Can you go get the paperwork up to date?" Implying because the shift doesn't finish the person can do the paperwork although there is no real link between the two.

In ordinary conversation people don't often work from observable to non-observable, or from not in a specific trance to in a specific trance (some good communicators do). Normally it is just truism-suggestion, sometimes they can be linked but most people don't realise they are doing it so just use single sentences.

Another one could be:

- "You know where Johnny is? Can you call him for tea?"

In sales

- "Take a look at this phone; it meets all of your needs."

- "You look like someone that likes making good decisions; this is the TV for you."
- "You want the Big Mac Meal, and that is large." (Question said as a statement)

On TV

- "The question is shown on the screen; phone in if you know the answer."
- "It's the end of the show; enter this competition to win £5000."

What I am doing here is writing these keeping them as much as possible to just a single language pattern, so the sentences don't necessarily all sound as natural as they would if you say them mixing language patterns.

## Contingent suggestions

Contingent suggestions make one part of the suggestion contingent on the other. One part happens because of the other part of the suggestion. In reality the two parts don't have to link, it only has to sound like it links. You can link unrelated sentences and make them seem related. You usually link one part to the other with an active term like 'as, during, while, before, after, when'.

For example:

- "Take a look at this book as you think about what you want."

You can work from conscious to non-conscious or from observable behaviours to non-observable behaviours, or from external reality to internal reality, or you can simply work from a truism then link with a statement.

An example for problem solving might be:

- "When you see someone smoking, you can think about how good you feel that you moved on from that old behaviour."

As with the compound suggestions you want to pace and then lead

- "As you're sitting there with your legs crossed, your mind can begin to wander."
- "Don't allow the eyes to close until your unconscious mind lets you try to lift your hand."

Example of contingent suggestions:

- "You are reading this book as you hear your internal dialogue."
- "As you hear your internal dialogue you can be curious about what you will be learning."

- "Before that curiosity can deepen into unconscious learning you can read to the end of this chapter."
- "Don't let full unconscious learning happen until you have finished reading."

Some examples of contingent suggestions you may hear in everyday situations:

- "You don't have to brush your teeth until you're about to go to bed."
- "When you go to the shop remember to get some milk."
- "Wash your hands before you eat dinner."
- "I'll read you a story when you're in bed."
- "You can have chocolate fudge cake after you have finished your dinner."

Contingent suggestions make one part of a sentence contingent on the other. The way to word them is to ideally have the contingent part as a non-conscious process. If it is non-conscious the client can't say "no" when the behaviour it is linked to is true and happening.

- "As you blink in that special way you can become more absorbed."

- "As you breathe out you can relax deeper."

- "As you look at me, you can also be aware of certain thoughts that come to mind, as you become aware of those thoughts you can wonder what is happening in those hands, as you wonder what is happening in those hands you can notice that one hand feels different from the other…"

All of these pace and lead and all start with a truism, the first person is blinking, the second person is breathing out, the third person is looking at me. The contingent parts are all out of conscious control. Becoming absorbed, relaxing deeper, having thoughts, wondering what is happening in the hands, hands feeling different from each other. Nominalisation obviously helps here with the leading parts.

# HYPNOTIC LANGUAGE PATTERNS: PRESUPPOSITIONS

Presuppositions work like post-hypnotic suggestions. As you are repeatedly presupposing specific outcomes you are setting up future responses. If the responses that are being set up are associated with a behaviour that will definitely happen then this also increases the likelihood of the suggestion being followed.

Presuppositions are where you presuppose an outcome using terms like when, after, while, during, as, before. They are useful for making someone think along certain lines and can also be useful for setting up ideas for the client to think about which builds up a future of having that outcome. Sometimes immediately directly presupposing can seem too intrusive or pushy. Sometimes it can be better to start a sentence in a way that sounds harmless. Like starting a sentence with the word *would* or starting it applying to a third party.

Some examples of presuppositions:

- "Have you ever been in a trance before?" (Before the one they are in/going into)

- "While your unconscious mind works at creating the changes that you desire you can begin to relax." (While – implying that this is happening)

- "What would it be like if you discovered that when you wake up tomorrow that old problem is gone; what will be the first thing you notice?" (Starting non-threatening with "would" then moving to "when" implying that the problem will be gone and "will" implying there will definitely be things to notice)

Presuppositions are just where you imply something without saying it (like saying "try not to forget what I say" which implies it will be difficult to remember and so probably will be forgotten, or "have you been in a trance before" using "before" implies either before the one they are in now or the one they will be going into).

Presuppositions are where you are making an assumption that something will be happening. This can be done overtly or covertly. For example, if you say "how would you like to go into hypnosis today?" you are implying the client will go into hypnosis. You are expecting it. All you are asking is how that will happen not whether it will happen or not. With this specific question there is a chance that they could interpret the sentence literally and say that they would or wouldn't like to go into hypnosis today. The therapist is being curious about the how or when rather than whether something will happen. Presuppositions are a great way of keeping focused on curiosity. The therapist is assuming that change is inevitable, or success is inevitable. The only question is how and when. It is a question of when something will happen, not whether something will happen.

# HYPNOTIC LANGUAGE PATTERNS: VAGUE LANGUAGE

**Nominalisations**

Using words which are non-specific lead people to have to search internally for meaning (trans-derivational search). This makes those non-specific words sound meaningful to most people as they find their own meaning. It is useful to use nominalisations and other vague words and terms regularly, especially where you don't know something. They are words that the person has their own meaning for.

Nominalisation is using words with no fixed meaning like:

Curious, wonder, development, relaxing, explore, resources, pleasure, excitement, enjoyment, discover, fun, relax, meets your needs, satisfaction.

Negative nominalisation can be used as a way of describing the problem even if the therapist doesn't know all the details, if they use the term anxiety the client will know what they are talking about even though the therapist may not really know what it means to the client. If the therapist then talks whilst leaning to look behind the client whilst mentioning anxiety, for example, and put it in past tense by saying something like "the old anxiety" can place the problem in the past. They can also alter the meaning of a nominalisation, so they could start with *anxiety* and the client's meaning and begin to reframe and alter the meaning of the nominalisation so that when the client thinks of *anxiety* it has a different meaning to them now compared to the meaning it had before the session. I worked with an alcoholic. He kept saying it is his addiction. This was how he phrased it. He had his own meaning for what he meant by the phrase "it is my addiction". I ended up reframing the idea of addiction as being bullied and pushed around and compared it to an abusive relationship.

Following this, when he would talk about it being his addiction he would think about it as him being bullied and in an abusive relationship and he would get angry at the thought that he was letting himself get bullied and abused which motivated him every time he thought about it to take action against it. Weeks later he was proud to tell me he was no longer a victim to his addiction. Or the therapist could begin to change the nominalisation used and start using a different one, building up different meaning for this nominalisation and for the problem. For example, if someone is talking of being in pain, the therapist may bring in the term discomfort rather than the word pain as they talk about the pain, so that they begin to use the word discomfort, or identify with the word discomfort (which has 70% of its letters spelling comfort). I used this for a client in pain. I began using the word discomfort rather than pain, they gradually started following along with this using the word themselves when talking about the pain, then I explained how 70% of discomfort is comfort which had multiple meanings. It is a truism, 70% of the word is the word comfort, but in relation to them now thinking about their pain as discomfort I was saying that 70% of that discomfort was comfort which led to a decrease in the experienced pain.

Another area with therapeutic nominalisations, is building your own context through the links between the nominalisations. If *development* was used with talk of business the meaning of development to the listener is more likely to be in the context of business and it could be good or bad. If *development* was used in the context of "what is happening now?" then it is more likely to bring up meaning in this context and *development* in a personal coaching session is likely to have the person assume it is associated with their personal development.

The context the nominalisation is given in impacts on the meaning of the nominalisation.

"New developments are happening in the business, there will be organisational changes and improvements taking place."

"New developments are happening in your life, and these may lead to organisational changes and improvements taking place giving you more time for yourself."

"New developments are happening inside your mind, and you can wonder how those organisational changes and improvements will take place."

## Suggesting direction but not the way

Nominalisations can be used to aid the client non-consciously to begin to spread change to other areas of their life. For example, I had a single therapy session where I worked with a woman that over the phone said she wanted to quit smoking then came to me and said she wanted to lose weight and stop drinking cola and quit smoking. I asked which one of these was most important to her. Quitting drinking cola was what she expected to find hardest and was most important to her. I helped her with this issue whilst dropping in nominalisations and non-specific ideas for change in other areas to also occur. She lost about a stone and a half in less than three months, cut down on smoking and had no problem stopping drinking cola with no side effects. My aim was to promote a way for her non-consciously to spread change and apply the therapy to all these areas, not just the area I was mainly focusing on helping her with. Asking things like "You can be curious to discover what other changes occur." A sentence with no specific meaning other than the one the listener places on it and it doesn't give any direction or content as to what is expected other than change. Given in a context where all change that is happening is positive the expected change is also likely to be positive.

## Using vague language during inner experiences

When people are entering hypnosis, or perhaps are following along to an induction, one of the most jarring things a therapist can do is to suggest something that doesn't match the experience the client is having in their mind. When hypnotising people or guiding their inner experience the therapist can talk about "I wonder whether there are any clouds in the sky and what they look like." This statement is vague, if there aren't clouds in the clients' inner experience that is fine, if there are and the clouds are stormy, that is fine, if there are light wispy clouds that is also okay. If the therapist says "and you can see that clear blue sky." they may be wrong, the sky in the client's mind may be dark and stormy so this suggestion can be jarring and can interrupt the flow of their experience. If the therapist knows information, like if the client has said about a stormy sky, then this can be said specifically as the therapist knows it is true. If the therapist doesn't know then it is best to be curious about what the client is experiencing, like I mentioned above about clouds. If the therapist wants something specific in the clients' experience then the therapist can suggest the discovery of it rather than directly saying it is there, like saying "I wonder whether (or when) you will notice the stream and when you become aware of that stream just take some time to drift deeper into the experience." By being curious the therapist is guiding and narrowing the client's attention on having them noticing what their own inner experience is, without dictating to them what they have to experience.

**Naturally hypnotic language**

Using vague language is naturally hypnotic. When vague language is used clients have to find out what the therapist is talking about. To do this they go on an internal search for meaning to create their version of what the therapist is saying so that they can understand it. An everyday version of this is politician speak, for example; "You have all come here today to listen to what I can do for you and I will make all those changes to education you know need to be made, I will make those big decision, those tough decisions, doing what the other party has failed to do, because it is what you want, it is what we want, and it is what is right."

None of this means anything, but at the same time it means almost everything. Every listener that cares about education and feels that there are certain tough topics that never seem to get addressed with assume that the speaker is talking about those issues.

**Multi-level communication**

By using vague language, the therapist can talk about a range of different topics and keep bringing up the same vague terms or terms with multiple meanings as a way of getting certain ideas across. The therapist can seem to talk about how a gardener knows when it is time to harvest vegetables from the vegetable patch, and then talking about how a singer knows how to breathe correctly for any given song and actually be mentioning how the client can relax in situations that previously made them anxious.

**A Collection of Positive Nominalisations & Ambiguous Statements**

- Express the true you
- Positive qualities
- Purpose
- Meaning
- Following your heart
- Self-realisation
- Self-discovery

- Authority
- Leadership skills
- Top dog
- Management qualities
- Taking opportunities for success and achievement
- Use your strengths to achieve success
- Charisma
- Respect
- Love
- Connection
- Special feeling
- Community
- Togetherness
- Meaningful

# Hypnotic Language Patterns: Binds

A bind is where you offer more than one choice with the same outcome. For a bind the choice can be consciously chosen. You give people illusory conscious choice. They can pick which response they want to follow. They also have the option of rejecting all choices.

For example:

- "Would you like to sit in the left or the right chair to go into hypnosis?" (Implication is whichever chair they chose to sit in they agree to go into hypnosis)

Binds are of great use to therapists because as they appear to offer choices they make the client feel that they are in control because they are choosing while the whole time all choices only have one outcome. If the therapist uses a double bind they presuppose one direction whilst the client thinks they are always making the choices.

## Illusion of choice

All binds offer an illusion of choice. The therapist is offering different options that lead to the same or similar outcomes. What clients focus on is the choice point, not the implication, or outcome. If the therapist suggested "do you think the left hand or the right hand will lift as you go into hypnosis, the client's attention is focused on which hand they think will lift, and they can even say neither hand (and this response can be linked into the double bind), yet all the responses lead to a single outcome of going into a trance. The question is about which hand they think will lift. Not a question of whether they think they will go into hypnosis. If they say they think the left hand will lift, they are saying they think it will lift as they go into hypnosis. If they say they think the right hand will lift, they are saying they think the right hand will lift as they go into hypnosis. If they say neither hand will lift, they are saying neither hand will lift as they go into hypnosis. What isn't in question is that they will go into hypnosis. The only question is whether they are right or wrong. They may say the left hand and the right hand might lift, or both hands may remain stationary as they go into hypnosis and so they may be wrong about their choice of hand, but this doesn't change the outcome.

## Consciously answerable binds

A bind on its own is consciously answerable. If a therapist says to a client "do you want to sit in this chair or that chair to go into hypnosis?" the client can decide about which chair to sit in to go into hypnosis. They can also refuse to sit in either chair, in which case they won't be going into hypnosis.

## Double binds

Double binds are a class of language pattern where the therapist offers choices to the client but it doesn't matter which choice they follow the outcome will still be the desired one. With double binds the outcomes are often non-conscious so the client has little chance to sabotage it, and the bind options are more about noticing, or discovering rather than actively choosing the goal. Whereas a bind is a conscious choice which can easily be sabotaged.

Bind: "Do you want to sit in this chair or that chair to go into hypnosis?"

Double Bind: "I wonder whether you will sit in one of the chairs, stand up or do something different as you go into hypnosis?"

The bind can be ignored by standing up or lying on the floor or just flatly deciding "I'm not going into hypnosis."

The double bind leaves it open for almost any response to occur for the person to enter hypnosis. "Do something different" could mean almost any response; and "as" being used instead of "to" means it is going to happen the question is what will they be doing whilst hypnosis is developing.

Some more examples of double binds:

- "I wonder whether you will you go deeper into hypnosis with the sound of my voice or the spaces between my words?"

- "Which hand do you think will lift as you enter hypnosis or do you think neither hand will move?"

- "Do you think that left hand will get warm first or will it be the right hand?" (Implication is that one hand will get warm then the other. They can say which hand they *think* will be the first to get warm. They could be right or wrong. All they are asked is for their opinion on what response they will give first)

- "I wonder whether you will go deeper into hypnosis with the sound of my voice, or will it be with each out breath that you take?" (Implication that they will go deeper into hypnosis; and that they are already in hypnosis. They have to wait to discover if it will be my voice or their breathing that takes them deeper)

The outcome is to get a non-conscious response

- "You can forget to remember the things you forgot or remember to forget the things that you remember." (A double bind for amnesia)

- "You can be curious about a rigidity in that arm without being aware of it, or aware of the rigidity in that arm without paying it any attention' (A double bind for catalepsy)

- "I don't know whether you will see what isn't there, or believe that you see it without being able to see them?" (A double bind for hallucinations)

- "I don't know whether you will discover an hour of hypnotic time can seem like a minute, or you can discover a minute of waking time can stretch into an hour." (A double bind for time distortion)

- 'I don't know whether you will drift back into a pleasant memory unaware of the future, or discover yourself in the memory curious about what the future holds?" (A double bind for regression)

- 'You can be aware of that hand unaware that it is yours, or know it is your hand but be unaware of it." (A double bind for anaesthesia)

## Selection of examples of different types of binds

- "I don't know whether you will decide not to stop smoking until the end of the session or decide to stop smoking before that."

- "It's easy to forget how easy it was to remember that you smoked, while finding it hard to forget how easy it is to remember many happy memories."

- "I don't know whether your unconscious mind will keep your mouth closed if you try to smoke, or if you try to put a cigarette in to your mouth you will discover that it won't open."

- "I don't know whether you will enjoy life more because you no longer smoke or whether it will be because you have cleaner lungs?"

- "Will the memory that comes to mind be a motivated one or will it be a memory of high motivation?"

- "Will you maintain a cleaner and healthier lifestyle to prove to others how capable you are or will it be to prove it to yourself?"

- "You may get a temporary craving over the next few days, I wonder whether it will be your extra energy that fills that craving or will it be that smile that is showing your pleasure you have because of your success?"

- "Will you decide honestly and unconsciously to show people that you are proud of whom you are or show them that you are proud of whom you have become?"

- "I wonder whether you think that you will be aware of making that unconscious choice to permanently stop smoking now or whether it will just happen without your awareness?"

- "There are times you can remember when you forgot what you tried to remember, there are also times you can remember when you forgot what was in your mind only seconds ago, remembering that you forgot to try to remember what it was that you forgot, like now finding that you remember you will forget if you try to remember but knowing that you have forgotten what you didn't try to remember, forgetting why you're even trying when you know you will just forget everything that I have said but knowing it is not forgotten unconsciously."

There are many types of double binds. If you learn what is in this chapter and follow the fundamental principles you will automatically be doing the different double binds. Once you feel confident with the Ericksonian approach it can be worth exploring the language patterns further to help to refine your skill and enhance your knowledge. There are double disassociation double binds, conscious-unconscious double binds, reverse-set double binds, time binds, and non-sequitur double binds (Erickson & Rossi, 1976).

# HYPNOTIC LANGUAGE PATTERNS: COMMANDS & SUGGESTIONS

### What are commands and suggestions?

My view is that commands are telling someone what to do or having authority over someone, whereas suggestions are giving ideas or saying something in an indirect way. Commands can seem more assertive and so if someone isn't keen on being told what to do they may not like it and may not respond well to the command. Whereas suggestions can feel more comfortable as the therapist is offering ideas about how something can be done and not necessarily telling someone how to do something. They may also be more indirect and so be giving a fairly direct idea but in an indirect way to allow the person to do things their way rather than the therapists.

### Direct commands

When offering direct commands, a therapist will directly tell clients what they are to do, when and how and what they recommend the client does.

### Indirect commands and suggestions

These are a part of the Interspersal technique. Marking commands or suggestions as separate from the sentence with either a tonal shift or maybe by pausing before and after the command or with a specific gesture or movement etc. This causes a pattern that the non-conscious picks up on and responds to.

For example:

- "Some people find they...*relax deeply*...in the shower other people find they...*drift into a dreamy state*...when they are in the bath." (Indirectly suggesting *relax deeply* and *drift into a dreamy state*)

- "I don't know whether...*you will discover*...that...*you relax deeply*...as you listen to my voice...or whether ...*you will* *discover...*that...*you become more fully absorbed in your internal experience with each out breath...*" (Indirectly suggesting *you will discover, you relax deeply, you will discover, you become more fully absorbed in your internal experience with each out breath*).

Embedded commands and suggestions are where you are marking out a part of the communication for the client to pick up on and respond to non-consciously. This could be done with a gesture, with a head movement, with a tonal shift or a touch. As long as the marking out is done consistently the client will non-consciously pick up on it.

Some example of embedded commands could be:

- "Someone asked the other day how...*you go into hypnosis*...I began explaining to them the process of how...*you go into hypnosis*...I explained that firstly the client will be looking at me while I talk to them and probably won't notice at first how...*the breathing begins to slow down*...and as they...*begin to relax*...I continue talking to them and they...*go into hypnosis easily and effortlessly*..."

- "I remember travelling on a plane and discovering how high up we went...it was so difficult not to just...*close your eyes and fall asleep*...with the sounds in the cabin and the lights turned down...I couldn't help myself...*drifting off*..."

Embedded commands are used positively and negatively in everyday situations

For example:

Doctors or dentists telling you "this will hurt".

People telling children "you're never going to amount to anything, you're rubbish at maths" or "one of these days you're going to get hurt doing that".

Doctors telling the patient "the problem will last for three to six weeks".

To children "you're going to be so successful when you grow up".

Analogue marking is the process of marking out suggestions, ideas or communication; this helps the therapist to offer communication that is multi-layered. The client generally will consciously follow along to the bigger picture, to hearing the whole communication, while non-consciously they will recognise the patterns being conveyed in the communication.

It is important to be continually allowing communication to both the client's conscious awareness and to the client non-consciously. Analogue marking allows the client to consciously follow along to the communication whilst non-consciously they are aware of the marked-out sections. Because the client non-consciously notices these sections and consciously doesn't, it is like they receive two different messages. I often do this by telling stories or metaphors that the client can consciously listen to while they non-consciously responds to the patterns in what I am saying and also to any sections that get marked out (a form of analogue marking is embedded commands/suggestions).

The *My Friend John* technique developed by Milton Erickson (Erickson M. H., 1964) is a good example of this used in trance induction. It also happens in everyday life, you get people that say "I told him...*I'm really annoyed at the lack of respect you show me...*" As you hear someone talking directly at you like this it can feel like it is aimed at you, it creates feelings in your body as it affects you on a deeper level even though logically and consciously you know they are not talking about you (although they could be using this technique, and so they are talking about you, and they are hiding the message in a story to indirectly tell you they are annoyed at your lack of respect).

If ideas and suggestions are given indirectly (via analogue marking for example) then the client is highly unlikely to consciously notice, so it will only be received non-consciously. If the suggestions were given directly then the client may consciously become aware and may in the future sabotage the work. When I want to educate someone in therapy and feel that they probably don't see that they don't know what they don't know I do it indirectly. Often by telling them I'm not going to tell them because I am there as a therapist and they have come to me for help there is a high chance that they expect me to know what I'm talking about so if I don't give them reason to challenge me then often what I say gets accepted.

As an example in smoking, some people think they know the risks of smoking but don't really, they only know the common few things that get plastered over the media. I want them to understand some of the other issues that they have perhaps never really thought about or considered, but I don't want to lecture them or to have them defend why it won't happen to them (I don't always feel this is necessary, it is client dependant). I will often say "I know you know all the effects of smoking, so I don't need to tell you that 50% of all smokers die of a smoking related illness...etc." Then I tell them what I said I wasn't going to tell them but the way it has been introduced means they rarely challenge what I am saying.

To make embedded commands as effective as possible the most important thing is to do them so that the client doesn't consciously notice and to be consistent with how you do the commands so that the client can non-consciously pick up on the pattern.

Every person is different. Talking quickly can cause confusion and allow you to embed commands and use language patterns then move on before they have time to analyse it. Or you could talk with a broken rhythm or even just talk *normally* but add emphasis to the words you want to embed with either a movement, gesture, look, tonal shift with your voice or any other marker that can be picked up non-consciously by the client.

If you use shock or confusion inductions or techniques, you want to give clear direct suggestions so using embedded commands at these times isn't often the best approach at because the client will come out of hypnosis before you've used enough for them to notice the pattern. Following a shock or surprise induction you want to give them an escape from their confusion. To do this you need to give clear suggestions like saying "sleep" followed by continuing to give clear communication, like saying "that's right, now just allowing yourself to go deeper and deeper into hypnosis... and I don't know how you will choose to go deeper, whether it will be with each out breath or with the words I say or with the spaces between my words..."

# Hypnotic Language Patterns: Metaphors

Telling stories and anecdotes either mirroring the clients' situation, laying down a useful pattern, seeding or priming something for future work can be really effective in therapy. The therapist can set up a specific emotion with a metaphor or perhaps use client's comments or metaphors for rapport or use metaphors to lay down patterns non-consciously in the client. A story about circling a fort held by an evil invader, not letting food or water get in to the fort and not letting the invaders escape, after a short while all the invaders die could be used to fight warts, verruca's or even perhaps help with cancer treatment.

Metaphors are probably one of the most powerful techniques. There is the story I have mentioned previously of Milton Erickson teaching a boy who used to wet the bed about muscle control by talking about baseball (which is needed for baseball and controlling the bladder). Ideally the story or metaphor will be something that will come from the client and something the client can relate to. The story needs to be absorbing and acceptable. Metaphors, stories and examples are a useful tool in hypnotherapy because they allow the therapist to prime for things to take place. For example, if the therapist wants to elicit an arm levitation they can prime it in advance by talking about being desperate to politely get attention in class at school or reaching up to put shopping away or hailing a taxi or stopping a bus. All of these stories seed or prime the client with the idea of arm levitation making them more likely to do it as those patterns in the mind are activated.

If the therapist wanted to help someone forget pain they could talk to them about being in a cinema and needing the toilet as they enter but getting so engrossed in the film they forget they need the toilet. Or having fun playing as a child and not noticing any bumps and bruises or cuts until later when they are home. Again, these stories then activate related neurological processes. Stories also allow the therapist to lay down future useful patterns. If the answer to the problem is to be patient the therapist can tell a story that gives this message. If the answer to a problem is to relax they can lay down this pattern. They can be as abstract or as literal as they like. They could lay down a *relax* pattern by talking about a stick floating on a river that gets wider and wider and as it does the water slows down and isn't as rough and the stick floats slower and more gently. Or they could talk about a friend that had a situation at work that really was annoying them and how they overcame this. This second option would mirror the situation with a *recognisable* alternative way of handling things. They can also talk about past successes they have had with other clients in similar situations and what those clients did to move on.

### Patterns

A metaphor is just a pattern or template that can be taken, understood and used by the client non-consciously. It's about using the clients' language. The client doesn't necessarily interpret the content it takes the raw patterns from the metaphor and sees how this applies to the current situation. In the same way that a dozen very different crime novels may share the same underlying pattern, the presenting problem and solution is only one story on a pattern which many other stories can be overlaid onto. When reading a crime novel, most people don't notice that the structure is the same as the previous stories by that author and the same as dozens of other novels. To notice that they have to go beyond the content. It isn't that the reader was unaware of this as a being, they were just unaware of it because they weren't focusing on it. It doesn't take much questioning of a reader to elicit that they were aware on some level, especially with regular readers of the same type of stories.

**Generic metaphors**

When a therapist doesn't know what to do with a case, or quite what the answer or way forward is, generic metaphors can be helpful. Generic metaphors can also be helpful when working with groups or more than one person at a time. For example I worked with a group to test this idea and ended the group training by saying that one of them had something they wanted help with but didn't get a chance to have me help them with it, I said I know who they are and what that problem is and what help they need, but also respect their privacy so will tell them a story that is specifically for them, everyone else can just relax and enjoy the story, but you (the person with the problem) will understand how this relates to you and how this can help you to move forward, even if you don't understand that now or consciously. I then told a generic metaphor that had many patterns in it but wasn't actually targeted at any specific individual in the room, and over the months following this experience many of the course participants contacted me to thank me for the metaphor I gave them personally and told me how it had helped them. Each individual assumed the metaphor was for them and they found the meaning they needed, even though it wasn't actually aimed at anyone specifically.

## Client generated vs therapist generated

Our language is full of metaphors, from saying "he is a pain in the neck", or "I've been feeling blue", or "I feel trapped in a rut", or "the news hit me like a sledgehammer", through to more rounded and detailed metaphors. When the metaphors that the therapist uses for treatment have come from or have been developed from what the client has said they are often more impactful and effective. If a client talks of a stabbing pain of a headache, the therapist could talk of blunting that pain, or shielding that area from the stabbing, and these would be likely to be more effective than talking about numbing that pain. Or if a client spoke about feeling trapped (when talking about a specific situation) then the therapist can talk about finding a way out, escaping or some other *trapped* related solution, they can tell metaphors or stories about someone that is trapped and escapes, and this would be more helpful than perhaps telling metaphors or stories about gaining a new perspective or some other solution.

## Using metaphors to package suggestions, commands and ideas

As mentioned around commands and suggestions, metaphors are a great way of packaging suggestions and ideas. Some of this packaging as mentioned can be metaphorically laying down patterns, like telling a story of someone walking through a forest and then coming to a mountain and noticing there is a cave high up in the side of the mountain and so climbing and struggling up the mountain to get to that cave and then looking out from the cave and getting a new perspective on the forest below, can lay down a helpful pattern for undergoing therapy to get to a place where the client can look back and have a new perspective on the problem, and this metaphor can be carried forward to having other answers and solutions.

The therapist can tell a story and embed suggestions within the metaphor, below is an example of a story of snow white that was told to a team of staff in a care home.

The staff had begun to experience splitting, where staff that worked on different shifts began criticising staff on other shifts and blaming each other for things and had stopped working as a cohesive team. This story was told during a team day during a relaxation session to suggest the idea of working together as a team again:

One day Snow White decided that she wanted to go on a walk, she didn't often go out far from her home as she was unsure what she would find in the deep, dark forest. Snow White left on a path right outside her front door. The path was covered by trees arching high overhead; either side of her was deep, dark forest. Snow White stuck to the path walking through the shimmering beams of light that flickered down through the trees above. As she continued to...*follow this path*...she was aware of the rhythmic beat of her feet on the ground and the sounds of birds in the trees and the rustling of leaves as the wind blew a breeze. She continued to wander and at times found her mind wonder about why she set out on this journey...after walking for a while she found herself smile as she saw a house in the distance. The house was in a clearing in the forest that was bright and cheerful. There were plants of many varieties and many flowers surrounding the house. As Snow White reached the clearing she could feel the calm, warmth from the sun on her skin. Snow White could hear voices coming from the house and the closer she got the more she could tell that the people inside the house were disagreeing with each other. Snow White approached and asked one of the people what was wrong. Grumpy explained that they used to all go to work singing and dancing with enjoyment but now they seem to have forgotten how to *work as a team*. Grumpy explained that they used to push together...*pull together*...axe together...*all together*...but now they found that they couldn't. When one pushed another pulled and no work got done. Snow White asked what they do and was told that they are the team that digs and lays the foundations for new buildings. She asked them why they decided to do that work. She was told that you see buildings standing and feel proud because you know that they are standing because you built the foundations well, it makes you proud of all that hard work you did...Snow White decided to tell the little people a story about a centipede that kept falling over its legs. The centipede asked a friend how he manages to walk without falling over. He was told to just...*relax*...and let all the legs...*work together*...not keep thinking about which leg should do what and when. This made no sense to the dwarves so they decided to forget what Snow White said and just enjoy her company. Before Snow White left she asked who made such a lovely garden. The dwarves said they all worked at it and that many of the plants have survived some harsh winters. At the end of the day Snow White said good bye to the dwarves. She got right up and left. As she left she was amazed by how much happier and healthier they were starting to become. Something had happened that they were learning from which looked like it made them healthier and made them work out their differences, sneezy had stopped sneezing, grumpy was happy, bashful had clear skin and no hint of red, and all of the others had noticed improvements too. This made Snow White happy as she skipped away from the house up the path leaving her adventure behind like a dream that got more out of reach like a name on the tip of your tongue as she approached her home pleased with her mini adventure, then walked through her gate and, finding it was all a dream she...*opened her eyes...*

As you can see the character Snow White is me turning up to talk with all these staff, and in this story it starts talking about a journey and engaging the listeners in following the journey, as it continues it involves a home of dwarves mirroring the care home, there are embedded commands for working together, the care home was for teenagers, so the dwarves talk about what their job is, which is to lay foundations for new buildings, mirroring the care home staffs job of helping the teenagers develop the skills they need for adult life. There is a metaphor in a metaphor with Snow White talking about the centipede, this metaphor lays down the idea of working together without thinking about it, and without effort. As the story approaches the end Snow White comments on the garden which all the dwarves have helped to make nice, this is used as a way of knowing there are strengths there, and there are times that the staff will have worked together successfully, they perhaps just need reminding of those times and need the pattern for going back to working like that again reignited. At the same time, it is an opportunity to mention being able to continue to work together successfully even when things get tough. Then the story ends with ideas for inducing conscious amnesia by talking about the experience being like a dream or something on the tip of your tongue. I don't directly say forget this story; as that is one quick way of making people remember it. I wanted the staff to forget the story so that they wouldn't analyse and sabotage the ideas in the story. I wanted them to make positive changes non-consciously.

The story also ends with a description of some of the dwarves and how they are following things improving, and I linked specific individuals and traits with specific dwarves. I did wonder whether anyone would notice I was talking about them, but no-one seemed to notice. One of the staff had allergies so I had sneezy stopping sneezing, one member of staff was known to generally be grumpy and complaining, even when everyone got on well, so I had grumpy getting happy, and one person had eczema so I had bashful not being red-faced. I wanted to add something that let everyone non-consciously know that this whole story had been about them, I didn't want them to pay attention to that consciously though.

This story wasn't told straightaway, as mentioned, it was during a relaxation session, so I had been talking for a while guiding the staff into a relaxed place before telling the story but ended the experience with the end of the story. Having had that period of relaxation first helped to stop people being so likely to analyse what I was saying and so less likely to think "he's talking about me there" or "he's talking about them there".

Tasks that are given to clients can also be metaphorical. So, an alcoholic could be asked to look after some cacti as a way of teaching them about surviving without alcohol. Or someone with depression could be asked to find a stone on the beach, carry it around with them for a few weeks before revisiting the beach and throwing the stone in the sea as a way of teaching them about carrying around an uncomfortable problem and then deciding to let it go.

# Paradoxical Interventions

Within the Ericksonian approach one thing that is often used are paradoxical interventions. I find paradoxical interventions often develop naturally from applying the fundamental principles of an Ericksonian approach, I also don't think they are usually very paradoxical, just logical. An intervention is paradoxical when it seems like the opposite thing to do, or an unusual thing to do that for most people perhaps doesn't seem like it would work. Like suggesting to an alcoholic to drink alcohol or an insomniac to stay awake, or a teenager that is refusing to go to bed to stay awake as late as they can.

I have used paradoxical interventions frequently with people, here are some examples where I have used paradoxical interventions successfully.

I worked with an alcoholic, whose pattern was to go to buy three bottles of vodka, take them home to his flat and drink them there until he passed out, then repeat the process when he had sobered up enough to go to the shop to get more (normally the next day).

I had two sessions with him where he took no notice of anything, he had no intentions of changing yet his father had asked me to help him as he didn't know what to do. The man didn't ask for help himself.

It is easier to encourage someone who doesn't want to stop doing something to agree to do more of it so this is what I suggested. I told him that he obviously wanted to keep drinking and wanted to keep seeing me so that his father wouldn't kick him out of the flat (his father owned the flat, due to his drinking the man, who used to work as a lawyer was unemployed) but I'm not going to waste my time seeing him if he isn't prepared to work with me. I said I also didn't want his father to think that this was a waste of time, so would he agree to do some drinking that will let him explore his issues with drinking and learn something and at the same time he can tell his father that I told him to do it as an experiment.

He agreed. I told him what I wanted him to do was when he felt he needed a drink to go to the pub (which was closer than going to the shops where he normally purchased his vodka), order 3 pints of beer, line them up in front of him and gulp back the first one then say 'fucking therapist making me drink this beer', then gulp back the second and third pints doing the same, then go home. If he still wanted to drink more he was to go back to the pub to do the same again. He did this and stopped drinking on his own a few weeks later (I have done this type of intervention on a few occasions with alcoholics that drink alone at home and that don't drink beer).

I worked with a smoker that was referred to me by the NHS quit smoking clinic. He came in and said "I'm going to tell you what I told the lady that ran the clinic, I will have you smoking 50-a-day before you can stop me smoking 50-a-day".

He didn't come across as very motivated to quit, he knew all the reasons he had been told he should quit but said he didn't want to but he would see me and then he can tell everyone how he had tried everything. I saw him for a first session, by the second session he stuck to his word of ignoring everything and wanted to stay smoking, so again I told him I want him to try an experiment just so I know a bit more about his habit, and that it would involve him continuing to smoke at least the same amount as he does currently. He agreed he would do what I asked.

One of his patterns that happened every few days was that he drove to a supermarket to get food shopping. He didn't go to the nearest supermarket because he had to have a fixed number of cigarettes. He would have one when he got in his car, two on the journey and two in the supermarket car park (because he knew he couldn't smoke in the supermarket so he had to have extra before going in there). I told him what I wanted him to do was to wait until he got into the car park then smoke all five cigarettes and one more because he had to wait so long before having any. He enthusiastically agreed to do this thinking it sounded easy.

He cancelled his next appointment. I bumped into him in town a few months later. He said he was really angry with me. He did as I asked but he found that sitting in the car when he had shopping to do and *having* to smoke 6 cigarettes really annoyed him, all he wanted to do was get into the shop, get his food and go, but he was stuck outside the shop still smoking, he was resenting the cigarettes. He ended up deciding not to smoke in his car because of this. This then spread to forgetting to smoke after he was home out of his car and over a few weeks he was regularly forgetting to smoke and at the point I saw him he rarely smoked.

## Prescribing the symptom

One of the most commonly used paradoxical interventions is prescribing the symptom. Often therapists try to encourage clients to stop their symptoms, but even things we don't really like are difficult at times to let go of when we do them instinctively or they serve a purpose. It is much easier to get someone to agree to do something they already do than to try to get them to do something entirely new.

If someone has a habit of biting their nails perhaps it can be suggested they bite their nails more, or in a different order, or at a different speed. If someone smokes perhaps they can be suggested to smoke more, or in a different way. I think of it as being like *Chaos Therapy*. What the therapist is doing is finding a way to insert a small change that the client will accept into the pattern of the problem and using this as a starting point this creates a snowballing effect. What the therapist is doing is focusing on how they can change the pattern of the problem in some way so that a new pattern can take over. They just need to find that one thing which will unravel the problem and something which is such a small or simple thing that the client will have no problem taking it onboard and making that small change.

For example, cravings only last a few minutes even if at the time of a craving it can seem like it is going to last or feels like it does last for ages. Cravings also aren't usually as bad as they feel, it is just that there is nothing to compare the severity of it to. If a smoker compares a craving to the experience of a bad toothache they would usually agree they would prefer a few minutes of the craving. Without this comparison they may say they would virtually kill for a cigarette when a craving strikes. Because a craving doesn't last long in reality, if it is suggested to a smoker that when they get a craving would they be prepared to do relaxing breathing for one minute and if they still want a cigarette after that then they can have the cigarette. Most smokers are happy to do this, it is easy to do, but it can have a big impact on their smoking habit. Most people say one of the reasons they smoke is to relax, yet nicotine is a stimulant, it is the deep breathing smokers do and taking a break which helps them relax. So when they do that minute of relaxing breathing they can end up no longer needing a cigarette, they are also giving themselves some time so the craving may pass, something else could occur which distracts them and they forget to have the cigarette, so this one small change could disrupt their pattern and lead to them quitting smoking without any willpower or effort.

If someone is depressed and sits down doing nothing at home, maybe they can be encouraged to be depressed and sit down in a library doing nothing, with a book of interest in front of them open even if they don't read it, just so that it looks like they are reading. If they are able to do this and agree to do this they don't realise that the therapist has just increased the chances that someone will end up eventually striking up a conversation with them perhaps about the book and this conversation may be the beginning of socialising more again and focusing externally on other things rather than worries or negative thoughts and of getting their innate needs met.

The question is, what can be altered about the pattern that may seem insignificant or irrelevant to the client but which is something they are likely to agree to do that is likely to lead to a positive change in the future. This could be changing the frequency of the problem, the duration of the problem, the order the problem happens in, the location of the problem, adding in an extra element to the problem, or using the problem for something else. Problems can be made into chores, like having someone that can't sleep, agree to thoroughly clean their house all night long if they are still awake 15 minutes after going to bed. There are many different ways of intervening seemingly paradoxically. In the book on therapeutic trance-formation I will focus on different therapeutic approaches to helping people overcome their problems, including more on paradoxical interventions.

# HOW TO CRAFT HEALING STORIES

One of my favourite ways of working is through the use of healing stories. As has been mentioned in the chapter about metaphors, when working with clients to help them overcome their problems or to achieve success what the therapist is working with are the patterns for the problem not the content of the problem. Using stories allows the client to do therapy in their own way. It is a very client-centred way of working. All the therapist is doing is presenting the pattern for the problem and solution but leaving the client to find their own solutions. The therapist isn't dictating how the client should get better. Stories lay down, update and stimulate the client's neurological patterns, they allow the client to view their problem from an observing-self position rather than from within the problem. It is like rising up above a forest to see where you are and where you can go, compared to being in the middle of the forest only seeing dense trees.

Stories help to make something more memorable. If I present something like a story about not seeing the wood for the trees that will be more memorable than if I just say that people sometimes only see the problem from within the problem, what is helpful is for them to be able to get a different perspective on the problem. If I tell a client a story about someone struggling up a mountain, having different and interesting experiences during the journey up the mountain, perhaps defeating a dragon to make it to the top of the mountain and then looking out from the top of the mountain over the land and seeing how far they have come and how they have overcome various challenges, this will be impactful and memorable.

To tell an effective healing story the therapist needs to engage all of the senses. They need to be absorbing attention, which is essentially then hypnotising the client giving greater access to the inner potential of the client. Ideally stories will be based on things that the client has communicated, so if they said that their problem was like being stuck in a rut then the therapist may create a story around this idea meaning that the story resonates with the client, like having shared language and seems familiar to them. They also then understand on some level that the story is to do with their issue because the therapist is using metaphors and content they gave to describe the issue and challenges they are facing. If the client had commented about feeling stuck in a rut the therapist may talk about someone getting their car stuck on a mud track on a country road late at night in the pouring rain and struggling to get the car out of that rut. They would tell a story which would resolve the issue and get the car out of the rut and this pattern which was shared could then be applied to the presenting problem by the client to help them overcome the issue. The client may not do this with conscious awareness, it could be that they just find they start doing things differently in some way. Because the metaphors come from the client and the client doesn't have anything directly told to them about what they must do storytelling can bypass client resistance. It is hard to resist something when there is nothing being told to you to resist.

As has been mentioned many times in this book and the first *Hypnotherapy Revealed* book, *Introduction to Hypnotherapy*, the brain works like a pattern-matching machine and dreaming brain processes are largely like learning brain processes. Stories resonate well with how the brain works. In *Introduction to Hypnotherapy* I shared about the brain doing sloppy pattern matching and how this happens in a metaphorical way, this makes storytelling an obvious choice for a therapist to use in therapy because the therapist can present ideas metaphorically and the brain of the client will observe the pattern. Often what goes on consciously is very analytical, trying to understand things and usually looking at the surface details and content to find meaning. This isn't the same for everyone, but for many. Whereas non-consciously they will be perceiving the underlying pattern or structure rather than the overlaying content.

Storytelling has been used throughout history to help people through life transitions, to educate, to share moral teachings and to make information more memorable. Prior to written texts information had to be conveyed orally. It is easier to remember and share stories than cold information. Stories offer a disassociated, non-judgemental look at problems and allow clients to look at the pattern of the problem and solution from an emotion and content free perspective. This doesn't mean that the stories are emotion free, but what the client doesn't have is the emotional clouding which can happen when someone is absorbed in the problem. There may be emotion in the story which mirror or have some relevance to the problem, but they are part of the story and can be perceived in a way that is therapeutic for the client, whether associated or disassociated. The story has content but it is free of the content of the problem.

One of the most common questions I get asked is where do I find my metaphors to create stories around and how do I know what to talk about? I touched on this in the chapter on metaphors. I get most of my metaphors from the client. I have other ideas which I just like and frequently use as part of the types of stories I like creating, like using nature, but most of what I talk about in my therapeutic stories come from what clients have said. If a client talks about a rut then I may create a story around this idea. If they gesture away from their face while talking about the problem, or mention needing to get distance from their problem then I may create a story around the idea of gaining perspective. If, while talking, the client digs their heals into the ground I may tell a story about someone digging their heals in. If they rub their neck while talking about their relationship maybe they think their partner is a pain in the neck, so I might create a story around the pain in the neck idea. Metaphors permeate every aspect of our life. We use them almost continuously and often don't notice or realise that we are using metaphors, or that others are using metaphors because they are so common.

It is important to listen and observe for metaphors, especially getting used to common everyday metaphors, those phrases we hear all the time and overlook because everyone says them. These work well in therapy because we have a shared understanding of the metaphor. So I could create a story about a fat cat (or fat cats) for a client experiencing issues relating to their employment and perhaps changes in the workplace and this metaphor would likely be understood because they would understand about the metaphor of fat cats. The therapist should listen for words and phrases that clients use and also the client's actions, like digging heals in when talking about something they don't really want to change, or rubbing their neck when talking about their partner, or covering their eyes or closing their eyes when talking about something they don't want to face up to. Every client will have their own personal metaphors and will have their own personal interpretation or meaning for the metaphor to them. Sometimes problems themselves can be metaphors and then can be tackled by creating a story including the problem metaphor. For example, someone may present with a painful stiff shoulder where they have a *cold shoulder* because perhaps there is a relationship issue somewhere in their life where someone is giving them a *cold shoulder* and not talking to them. Maybe they have developed tingling in an arm or hand that feels like something is crawling under their skin and it turns out that something like a situation or person in their life makes their *skin crawl* and they have turned this phrase into a real experience. These metaphors can all be used to create therapeutic stories.

People may describe problems as burning, stabbing, sharp pain, need perspective, stuck in a rut, pain in the neck, feeling numb and many more descriptions. The therapist will be observing for all of these and looking at how they can integrate these into the therapeutic story they develop. They can also integrate observations about the environment or things they know about the client, like hobbies, interests, skills or life events or anything else which may fit well into a story making it more tailored and personal to that client.

My therapeutic storytelling process begins by asking the client what they would like to achieve. I want to know what goal they want, not what they don't want and perhaps a brief description of the problem in some instances. I listen and observe for metaphors and observe for the pattern of the client's situation. The content that they give may be helpful for metaphors and resources which can be used to help the client, but the pattern being presented will give the information needed to help the client to move on from the problem. Once I have the pattern I use this as the starting place for my story. This will be the structure which I build the story onto. Then I use the content, client metaphors and my own ideas to build up a story around that pattern. I may also use ideas from the environment and what you know about the client. I do this in real-time while talking with the client. I present the story by just asking the client to gaze off at something or to close their eyes, whatever is most comfortable for them. I take a few moments to help the client relax, get comfortable and focused on me as the therapist. Then I present the story and metaphors while closely watching the client and their reactions so that I can judge pacing and wording and change what I am doing and saying if needed. I don't pre-script anything. The client has given me all the information, all I am doing is recalling what the client has communicated and linking it together into a therapeutic narrative.

As I slowly and calmly tell my story I talk about what the client can see, hear, feel, taste, smell in the story. I use a mix of vague and specific language. I am vague when I don't know the specifics and specific when I do. If I want something specific in the story then I introduce it before it is needed as something for the client to discover and will carefully have them exploring to discover that thing I want them to have in their experience. Often this would be perhaps a hut, or a stream, or campfire, or tent, or bridge, etc. I use association for experiences within the story, often to have the client try out certain behaviours, thoughts or feelings, and disassociation for perspectives, where I want to have the client learn from the experience and gain perhaps gain a new perspective. Clients being associated during the story is often more of an emotional experience, whereas when they are disassociated they often have more of an analytical, observer experience.

When a therapist is starting out they are likely to be happy if they have been able to create one complete story. As the therapist becomes more experienced they can start to create multi-layered stories and metaphors to repeat patterns in different ways, or to present multiple patterns and to encourage amnesia. They can do stories within stories, or just be telling a single story, but draw in different metaphors or ideas which all have the same underlying pattern, or perhaps all address different problem patterns. I frequently use dreaming or a character in the story telling a story, or the main character having a flashback or flashforward as a way of introducing alternative stories or metaphors. When there are multiple metaphors or stories it is easier for someone to spontaneously develop amnesia about what took place in the middle of the experience. If a client was told a story which involved being out in the woods, and they sat under a tree and started daydreaming and imagining what it would be like to be on Mars, what is told to the client while they are imagining being on Mars is harder to recall after they exit hypnosis because it was sandwiched in the middle of the experience and memory is state-dependant so when the person is in normal wakeful awareness this is far removed from the deepest part of the story they were told. It doesn't mean that they will have amnesia, but it will be similar to a dream. If they focus on it and keep thinking about it then they will be more likely to recall it. If the therapist moves on and doesn't ask them about the experience then they will find it more difficult to recall especially as time passes.

Once the therapist has completed their therapeutic story they have to think about how they will end the session. I simply tell the client that they can drift back to the room in their own time. I want the client to feel empowered at all times. I want them to know that this is their experience and they are in full control of their experience. There are different ways that the story itself can end. The story can end with a specific conclusion, or the ending could bring the story back to the beginning. I like to make sure that the client drifting back to the room is contingent on them having made some therapeutic changes. I also generally don't encourage the client to analyse the story. If I think it would be helpful for them to analyse the story then I may encourage it, but generally I don't want them trying to analyse what we have done and perhaps undo inner work which has been completed. To reduce the client spontaneously analysing the story I may talk about unrelated things, or something I spoke to the client before therapy began, to re-orient their attention away from the hypnotic experience. I may also set tasks for the client to do which could include having the client do something connected with the story I told them that would then help to support the story in helping the client make changes in their life.

My biggest recommendation for those hoping to get more into healing storytelling is to start gathering stories in your mind, from books you read, to films, anecdotes and personal experiences. Learn different fairy-tales and other short stories which have endured. Those which resonate with you will stick with you, those that don't, which would need to be written down for you to remember them, they aren't stories for you. You want to be filling your mind with stories you like which resonate with you so that they come naturally to you when you share them. Then just practice telling therapeutic stories.

# THERAPY IN ACTION

### Therapy Session for Improving Artistic Ability

This is a transcript of a therapy session that includes my analysis to show what is going on to create change and to explain a little of what I am doing. In this session I am helping the client to improve their artistic abilities. I had looked at research into creating savant abilities in people (Snyder, 2009) and thought it may be possible to do this with hypnosis.

The session was from about 2005. It was an hour long and the only session required to help this client improve their artistic abilities and to still maintain and develop that improvement further as time has gone on (even at the time of writing this in 2018).

This annotated transcript has been included to demonstrate the Ericksonian approach in action. I use a 'D' for when I am speaking and a 'C' for the client. The analysis of what I am doing is *cut in* to the session where I have felt it is useful to note techniques or language patterns I am using. Hopefully this session will give a good overview of how the techniques and learnings from this book can be applied during therapy helping to bridge the gap between theoretical learning and practical application of hypnotic and therapeutic skills.

### Art Improvement Session

I ask the client to draw a picture of a horse in one minute and at the end will ask them to do the same again.

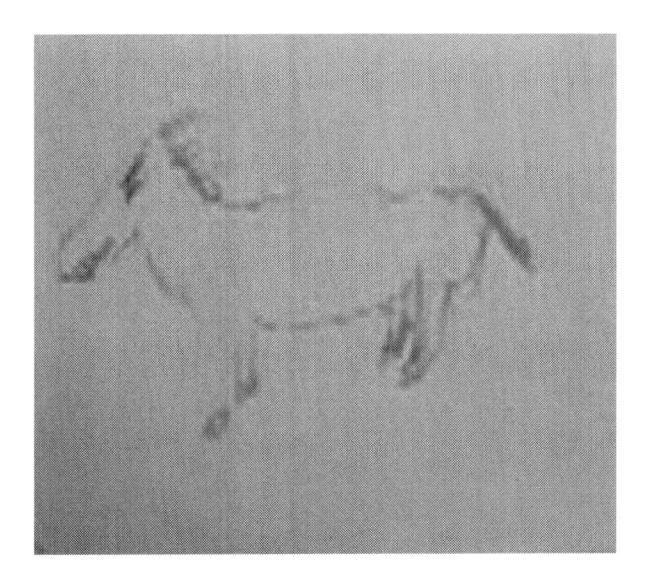

While this session was taking place, I was matching the clients arm positions, breathing, leg positions and leaning in at about the same angle the client is leaning back. This all helped with rapport and building a deeper connection with the client and their model of reality.

## Initiating Trance

> D: (Looking down from the client) When was the last time you (looking up at the client) *went into a trance*

C: Mmm... I don't know... probably in mmm, I went into a trance... well... probably last week... Tuesday... Tuesday this week because I was pruning my bonsai tree

D: When was the last time you (looking at the client in the same way I did above) *went into a deep trance...* (looking down) do you remember (looking back up at the client) *what one is like...*

C: Yep

D: *You do*

C: Vaguely

How I often start out inducing a hypnotic trance is by getting the client to recall a previous trance experience. If a client says they have never been in a trance before then I ask them what they think it will be like or what they expect it to be like; or I ask them about everyday trance states like leisure activities.

All the *italicised* words are embedded commands or suggestions. They are parts of the communication I am adding extra emphasis to by using a slightly deeper tone of voice, defocusing my eyes and relaxing my facial muscles all to imply trance through modelling what I am expecting.

I imply that the client has got experiences of entering a trance and deep trance by using the term 'when'; I don't ask 'have you ever been in a trance?' In some cases I may ask 'have you' if I strongly suspect they may not understand or realise that they have been in a trance before. If I do this I would use the term 'before' at the end of the sentence as 'before' implies either before the one they are in now or the one they will be going into.

I very often use feeding back as a way of embedding suggestions or commands; for example, when the client says 'yep' and I respond with the command 'you do'. I will often turn questions to statements with the tone of my voice. By feeding back what was just said you also begin to form a 'yes set' this is where you get yes responses that help to build rapport; displays understanding and makes it more difficult for the client to respond negatively to the work you do. If you get someone to say three or four yeses then give a suggestion you want them to follow they are more likely to do it than if you just gave them the suggestion on its own.

This client showed signs of not wanting to commit just yet by responding to my feeding back with the response 'vaguely' rather than responding by saying 'yes'. He had just answered my question by saying that he can remember what a deep trance is like but almost immediately became indecisive.

**Seeding/Priming Using Metaphor**

Sowing the seeds for amnesia and entering a trance when drawing.

> D: (starting to tell a true story to seed what is to come in the session, as I do I look down) You know when I was a kid I used to like watching...I can't remember the name of the programme now...that Rolfe Harris (turn to face the client) *drawing*... (keep facing the client but move my head position) kids programme that was on CITV...
>
> C: Rolfe's Cartoon Club
>
> D: Yeah something like that (I look down again) he used to have that like (drawing a

circle with my arm and finger) (looking back at the client) *circular desk thing*

C: (Doing an impression of Rolfe Harris)

D: (looking down again) And Mmm I (looking back at the client) *got the book of that* (Looking down again) I don't know how and I don't know what happened to it...it's not like me to lose a book...mmm...but I (looking back at the client) *always wanted to draw the Rolfaroo* (drawing in the air again)

C: Ahh yeah

I now use a true story to begin to plant the idea of automatic drawing. I also want the client to have amnesia for much of the session so that later they don't try to review everything that I was doing. This specific client has considerable experience with using hypnosis so I want to make sure they don't analyse the session too much when they come out of hypnosis. I also want to tell a story that lays down the pattern of the session we are in now where I want the client to start off more conscious, and then the unconscious can take over more. I also have chosen to use a story based on being a child of about eight years old because that way the client will begin to make associations unconsciously with when they were eight and this will cause a slight regression and will change the client's beliefs and opinions of what is possible; as an eight-year-old almost anything is possible.

I am still continuing to embed suggestions and ideas. While I am telling the story, I am drawing in the air (like automatic drawing taking place) and putting emphasis on the words I am saying while I do this so that the client knows that these parts are important.

> D: And in the book (gesturing where the book is) it tells you how to draw it, but I could never draw it, I could never get it to look like the one Rolfe Harris (looking at the client) *draws* (drawing in the air again)... (looking away) and I was 8 or something... didn't matter how hard I tried to draw it, it never looked like the ones Rolfe Harris draws...then one day I was in the lounge trying to *draw it* (drawing in the air)... kept failing, well not failing, I kept drawing it but not doing a good job... so I sort of gave up and still had the paper and still had the pen on me, and was watching something else, and then I thought 'yeah lets draw it again' (mimic going to

draw) (a car alarm goes off outside)... then I got distracted, by the TV... I can't remember what I was watching now but it distracted me and I suddenly thought 'cool I'll watch that'... didn't even think... It was one of those things where you know if you put an action movie on like Die Hard or something, and not a lot's happening so you're happy to read or do whatever, and then all of a sudden you hear some action happen and so you look up at the screen and think 'cool' and mmm so I looked up at the screen but my hand kept drawing... and I looked back down... and... like the cinema thing... you can be eating popcorn and something exciting happens and all of a sudden your hand freezes in front of your mouth because you're more concerned about (gesturing in front of me and looking in front of me – congruent – and gesturing holding a piece of popcorn in front of my mouth) what is going on, on the TV and all of a sudden that finishes and you carry on putting the food in your mouth (gesture doing this)... as if... you know... *the interruption never happened*...

and but what happened was my hand didn't stop, so when I was interrupted and I looked up, my hand continued to draw… and I looked down at a perfect Rolferoo and I was really proud except that it surprised me because I couldn't do it… (simulating trying to draw) never mind how hard I tried to draw it I couldn't draw it, and it took me by surprise because I did it without looking so I didn't know where anything was, so I shouldn't have been able to get the eye in the right place and I didn't know where the paper was… and people touch type and they can't see where all the keys are… they can get their fingers to the right keys… they can't see it at all… they can do it with their eyes closed and you know people play the piano the same… and people play the piano blind, like Stevie Wonder… so obviously it is possible for your body to know things that you don't know… like my granddad plays the piano without looking at the keyboard… and it is just one of those things… yes so Granddad can play the piano and not look at the keys… mmm could probably play

> in his sleep... and it's always fascinated me, I *can now*... I've never learnt to touch type, but *I can now* type to some extent without looking at the keys, as long as I don't consciously make the effort not to look at the keys, if I just glance up at the screen I can *keep my fingers going* (acting out typing without looking at my fingers) ... If I consciously think 'Oh I've been typing without looking at my hands' all of a sudden I'm pressing all the wrong buttons trying to type...

As the story continues I talk about how trying hard can lead to failure, or at least not getting the success you want. This is important because trying is a conscious process. And generally, the harder you try the harder something seems to become. In the same way that if you try to fall asleep you struggle and stay awake, and if you try to stay awake you fall asleep. What I want is for the client to just do, not try.

When a car alarm went off outside I decided to incorporate this into what I was saying so I spoke at that point of the distraction that gets your attention for a little while. I then continued to parallel the alarm by saying about an action film like Die Hard and hearing something happening that gets your attention. While I told this piece, I suggested amnesia and also suggested it being a positive distraction by interpreting the distraction in my story as 'cool'. I then talk about the hand continuing to draw while I am distracted partly because I want this process to happen in the client when he draws but also because if the alarm keeps going off or goes off again I want the client to be still responding on an unconscious level regardless of external distractions.

I create frustration in the story so that the client would become more focused on what I was saying. I spoke about how my hand continued moving then I ended that piece at an 'and...' before changing to talk about being in a cinema. What this does is a part of the client stays focused on looking for the completion of the pattern/story; and while that is happening the client enters a slightly deeper trance giving me the opportunity while they are partially listening and partially focused on waiting for the end of the story to continue to embed the idea of amnesia that I have been embedding already and also metaphorically commenting that the car alarm has stopped now.

I then carry on telling the story to convey the message that while the conscious mind is occupied with one thing the unconscious mind can work on something else. I then give different examples of being able to do things without conscious attention. Each example is true and undeniable which helps to convey the message that what we are doing is also possible. I use these stories to convey the message of not paying conscious attention, being pleasantly surprised by what the unconscious has done, which also contains the message that the conscious won't be a part of the process.

Towards the end of the story I start to separate conscious and unconscious by talking leaning slightly in one direction when talking about the unconscious mind and the other direction when talking about the conscious mind. I say '...it is possible for your body to know things that you don't know'. As I say this I spatially mark out; with my leaning; the body knowing and the mind not knowing.

I continue to seed the idea of doing things in a trance by talking about how my Granddad could probably play the piano in his sleep. I also suggest that conscious interference can stop this working just by having that conscious awareness; what is wanted is to just be in the moment and let it happen without thinking about it.

> C: That sucks yeah, but you're right you get similar sort of feelings like when you're trying

to draw or copy something and it doesn't do what it's supposed to do, I'd like to err, I don't know, say get a Disney video and be able to just put it on the side and just copy the video, that would be cool, I know people that can do that really, really, well and I can't understand why they can do it and I can't

D: Yes so it is possible obviously for your body to do things that you don't have an awareness of and obviously consciously you take in a certain amount of information, or at least you don't take it in, you take it in unconsciously and you're drip feed a certain little amount at a time and a very small amount of information, so you don't notice the fine detail, you don't really sort of, you just let the hand do what it is doing then it doesn't really matter what your conscious mind is thinking, what's on your conscious mind because your hand can just do it... any way that was just an aside... so you haven't been in a deep trance for a while?

C: No

In response to hearing my story the client agrees with what I have said and then states a goal that he would like; that would demonstrate success. He also says that he knows people that can do what he wants to do; which means he knows that it can be done. He also states that consciously he doesn't know how to do this; we are hoping to get him doing this without conscious awareness of how he does it; we just want him to do it.

My response to his statement was to focus on the unconscious process we are laying down and to link it back with him. He had spoken about 'other people' I wanted it to be him that has these abilities so I speak about his body doing things the conscious mind has no awareness of; again, I do this by marking out the conscious and unconscious so that when I talk to different locations he will know I am communicating with him on a conscious level or an unconscious level. I then very clearly state what will be expected; that he will notice fine detail and that what his conscious mind is doing has no relevance on his unconscious mind drawing as long as the conscious mind just lets it happen unhindered.

I use the term 'obviously' to convey the meaning that 'this is common knowledge, everyone knows this' this is to de-potentiate any resistance by using a term that is unlikely to be questioned. Generally, people don't question something that they feel they should know and they often just let it go in because you are not asking for a response. When I work with smokers I often do similar; I will say 'obviously you know all the dangers of smoking, so I'm not going to tell you that...' then I go on to list a load of dangers without receiving resistance because I have framed the statement as just telling them what I am not going to tell them.

## Induction

> D: There was something I wanted to do and the question is do I do it now or do I not? But I might give it a go...
>
> C: OK (looking confused)

I mention the induction I am going to do in this way as the client has been hypnotised by me before and I didn't want him to know what to expect. I wanted to begin to indirectly hypnotise him. The only way for the client to respond to what I said was for him to go inside his mind to wonder what I am thinking of doing and be confused because of not knowing what to expect. Most effective inductions have an element of confusion to disrupt the conscious mental set as the only way to respond to confusion is to try to find a way out; which will either be by following a clear suggestion by the Hypnotherapist or by going inside their own mind to escape the confusion.

> D: Mmm... only because it's just something different for a change...
>
> C: Nice day for a change...
>
> D: Yep I was just thinking exactly the same thing.... right put your hand on my hand... OK... in a minute I'm going to tell you to push down, now I don't want this to surprise you... so I'm going to tell you in advance what's going to happen...
>
> C: Alright

I mentioned 'something different for a change' so that the client would think of the sentence 'nice day for a change' which implies change happening. I also imply that because I am doing something different that will create the changes we will get in this session.

I tell the client what to do at the start of the induction I will be doing with him and even though I am about to do a very direct induction I still use indirect methods; I tell him I don't want the induction to surprise him and that because of this I will tell him in advance what will happen. I could have just told him directly 'when I do this you will go into a trance like this...etc.' but he may have chosen to resist me if I did that so by framing it that I am telling him for his benefit so that he knows what to expect he is more likely to listen to hear what is going to happen rather than feeling that he is being told what to do and feeling manipulated. I then change direction so that he doesn't have too long to analyse what I have just said in case he picks it apart and realises what I am doing. I don't just change to any old subject, I change to the issue of trance, getting some agreement, creating some confusion and again getting the client to recall a previous trance so that when I start the induction he is already partially in the recalled trance and mildly confused making him more receptive and has agreed with me a few times enhancing his receptivity and making him more likely to continue to accept what I say.

> D: And you don't mind *going into a deep trance,* do you?
>
> C: Nope
>
> D: You really don't mind?
>
> C: No

To make these sentences more powerful and less likely to be resisted I have used the reverse yes set. The reverse yes set is where you get a no but it is still in agreement with what you have said. By framing the questions negatively, the client is less likely to feel the need to disagree. By asking 'You really don't mind?' The client is likely to go inside their mind wondering is there supposed to be a reason to mind? So, this causes slight confusion for the client because why would they mind? While they are inside their mind searching previous trance experiences to make sense of the question and see if any previous deep trance experiences should lead them to a different answer they are putting themselves into a deeper trance just before I start the actual induction.

> D: What's the deepest trance you've been into? Maybe the one where you lost track of time, although you knew exactly what the time was because you came out of the trance at the right time... Right what I'm going to do is tell you to look into my eyes... not yet... so, what I'm going to do is tell you to push down on my hand (client starts pushing) in a minute... in a minute... (client laughing)... and... then when I say sleep (clicking my

fingers)... sleep... and do it your own way... you can go relaxed, feet up, head down, your choice, you can slump, do whatever you want, however you want to go into it... okay... *you happy with that.*

C: Yep

I then immediately ask 'what's the deepest trance you've been into?' And then begin to describe a trance experience suggesting that the client can go into a deep trance where he stops paying attention to conscious references like keeping track of time, where he can just be in each moment; and that he can come fully back when he is supposed to. I do this to keep the client occupied with thoughts of being in a trance. He is already partially recalling a trance experience from the last questions I asked; now he will be beginning to recall a specific deep trance experience.

I jump straight to describing what will happen with the current induction. All of this jumping around keeps some confusion there and keeps the client frustrated needing to become reliant on me for clues about what he is supposed to be doing. The client demonstrates that he is already becoming very receptive by responding literally to my description. He looks into my eyes when I mention it; and pushes down on my hand when I mention that.

> D: Right push down on my hand... really hard... push, harder, keep pushing, harder, harder, keep pushing harder, harder, push down harder, harder, look into my eyes, keep pushing down, harder and harder, harder and harder
>
> C: I can't?
>
> D: Keep pushing harder and harder, close your eyes and sleep...

This induction is a typical rapid induction. It is done very directly and forcefully. While I am doing this induction, I am closely watching the client. I am watching his face and shoulders looking for changes that will signal that he has gone inside his mind because it is at that point that I want to give the command to go inside his mind and sleep. After about 30 seconds the client says; just audibly; 'I can't'. It is at this point that I want to offer him a firm suggestion to sleep. When he says he can't he has almost given up trying; he has become slightly confused as how can he push harder if he is pushing as hard as he can. When people are confused they will usually accept any firm suggestion so long as it doesn't go against their personal values. In this induction that is when I say just once more 'keep pushing harder and harder' just to add to the confusion; then I say firmly and directly 'close your eyes and sleep' at the same time as clicking my fingers (which will trigger the reorientation response which is the response that gets fired to alert us to a stimulus making someone focus on just one thing; this fires as we enter dreams which is what can give the sensation of falling); I also pull my hand out from under his which also causes shock creating a trance state. With the shock from the click and from the hand being removed and with the confusion and the direct command the client was very unlikely to not go into a deep trance. The client slumps back into the chair as if all his muscles have relaxed and his arm falls to his lap.

**Trance Deepener**

> D: That's it, just allow yourself to go down deeper and deeper... that's it, deeper and deeper, just taking deep breaths, that's it... that's it...

I now deepen the trance very directly by telling the client to 'go down deeper and deeper' and saying 'that's it' on the clients out breaths. I also say 'just taking deep breaths' the reason for this was that by saying 'just' implies he is only going to take deep breaths not any other types of breaths.

> D: And in a moment I'm going to lift up that hand (looking over at the client's hands), and when I do I'm not going to tell you to put it down, any faster... that's it... than your unconscious mind begins...that's it... to get a sense of what it's like to walk down a flight of stairs...

I continue to frustrate responses to help continue to deepen the trance by being ambiguous; not telling the client which hand I will lift; by saying in a moment not specifying exactly when. I tell the client indirectly that I want him to do an arm levitation by telling him that 'I'm not going to tell you to put it down'. I follow this up with 'any faster' which implies that it will lower by itself (which as the sentence continues links the lowering with the unconscious walking down stairs).

I continue to say 'that's it' on each out breath by the client as I am still deepening the trance so I want to use everything to do this.

> D: And I'm not going to know where those stairs are... I'm not going to know whether they are in a building or whether they are going down to a garden... that's it... or down to a beach... *only you know*... that's it... where those steps are...

I emphasis me not knowing as this implies someone must know and if it isn't me it must be the client. I then tell him that he knows. I find that often it is best to indirectly imply something and lay down a pattern before saying something directly so that you are constantly communicating on two levels; one with implication and metaphor and patterns and the other being direct and able to be understood consciously. Even if I am talking to the unconscious mind I know the conscious mind is listening to some extent so it needs to have a message to follow that seems straight forward enough to not feel a need to analyse too much. Likewise, when I am talking to the conscious mind I know the unconscious is listening.

## Contingent Suggestions, Compound Suggestions & Nominalisations

> D: And the conscious part of you that is *normally* (emphasised) at the front of your mind can just distract itself in some way as you go down those stairs and it can find its own way of becoming more and more distracted with each step it takes

Contingent suggestions are suggestions where two parts of a communication are linked with an action phrase like; before, during, after, while, as. The two parts don't have to genuinely be linked or relate to each other. In the sentence above I link the conscious mind becoming more distracted with walking down the stairs in the mind even though there is no real link other than me saying 'as'. I also include a compound suggestion. Compound suggestions have two parts of a communication linked with an 'and' or a pause. They imply that because the first part happens so will the second part. In the sentence above I use 'and' to link the going down the stairs with becoming more and more distracted. In effect I am saying the same thing twice in the same sentence using two different language patterns.

In this sentence there is also the implication or presupposition that the client will be walking down the stairs and that he will be consciously distracted. The first half of the sentence was saying the conscious part can distract itself, the second half was about 'how' this distraction will happen. The idea behind this is that the client is now more likely to focus on the 'how' rather than whether the distraction will or will not happen. There is also the implication that the client is in a different state and things that happen in this state are different to normal waking state by emphasising 'normally' implying this isn't 'normally'.

There are also many nominalisations just in this one sentence. Nominalisations are words with no fixed meaning. The listener makes up their own meaning when they hear the words. From the start every session is full of nominalisations by the client and therapist. In the sentence above there is: normally; own way; conscious part of you; front of your mind; distract itself; those stairs (no description of the stairs); more (doesn't specify how much more so the client has to figure that out)

> D: And your unconscious mind that's *normally* at the back (separating conscious/unconscious with change in

> tonality, change in position my voice is coming from) can come to the front... and you can have an overwhelming sense of... *fully moving to the front*... with each step... that's it... and that unconscious part of you can... increase in awareness... of me of what I say... of the way that I say things... of tonality, subtle changes and can really... *fully become aware*... to the front of your mind...

Throughout the induction I am using the word 'and' to make sure that every part is linked. I am separating the conscious and unconscious as I talk to the client so that just by talking in a specific way and having my voice coming from a specific location the client will know whether I am talking to their conscious or unconscious mind or both. I am continuing to embed suggestions and commands to help the client's unconscious mind become more responsive to the way I am communicating to pick up on the marked-out communication; including communication that is targeted at the unconscious mind like metaphors and stories.

> D: Your conscious mind won't be completely to the back of your mind until you reach the tenth step... that's it... and the unconscious

part of you won't completely be at the front of your mind... won't *completely take over awareness* until you reach that tenth step and you can be curious to discover what is at the bottom of those stairs... that's right... that's right... (I lift up the right arm) and that arm can lower down only at the rate and speed that *you go deeper*... and you won't go all the way down into a deep comfortable trance state until that arm goes all the way down... that's it... all the way down... that's it... that's it... (the arm has lowered now)

The main purpose of the steps is as a deepener and to create greater separation between what is coming up which is the laying down of the patterns for improved artistic ability and the initial conscious thinking. Normally when people use steps they count the client down the steps. This relies on the client going at the speed the therapist sets. By doing the arm levitation I have a signal that I can visually observe that is linked to the client going deeper at a speed they choose. I continue to use negative phrasing saying 'you won't ... until...' this generally creates less resistance and is slightly harder for the client; especially when they are relaxed; to unpick and analyse.

Using negatives in this way people often hear the first part of the sentence (for example: You won't go all the way down into a deep and comfortable trance state) and if they are going to resist they often respond by doing it now and responding opposite to the statement. It is like a reverse double bind in that they can resist and respond now; or they can follow the suggestion and respond when they are asked to. The issue is about time not about whether they will do what they are being asked or not. It takes a lot for a client to then unpick the sentence and decide they will actually ignore it completely and not do anything. They are far more likely to choose - go against the therapist and do it now; or go with the therapist and do it when I am supposed to. Most people in therapy have made a commitment to be there to receive help so doing nothing when asked to is often not on their mind when they have an alternative to feel a sense of control and whatever other needs they would meet by going against the therapist.

> D: And you can wonder where you are going to wonder next... and somewhere there you can discover a painting... and I don't know what that painting will be of and what it is that *it can teach you something about yourself*...

Now that the client has reached the bottom of the steps I add a little confusion by using words that sound similar with one talking about thinking and one about action. I use many nominalisations as I don't know where they are going to be in their mind. And because I don't know where the painting that I want in their mind is going to be I don't tell them where it is; I give them the option to discover it. I keep using the word 'and' to continually compound end statement on the previous statement so that they build on each other. In many sessions I have observed people will say things like '...and in front of you, you will see a picture...' If the person can see in front of themselves in their minds eye before you have said that and there was no picture then you will mismatch their internal reality. By suggesting 'wonder and somewhere' it leaves the painting to be found. I also state a truism 'I don't know what that painting will be of...' This is undeniable with the implication that they must know. Being a truism, they again will agree with me. It is also followed with a poorly formed sentence. I run one sentence into the next using the words 'it can teach you' to transition from the end of a sentence with one meaning - saying ...what it is that it can teach you - then continuing the sentence giving a suggestion of what I want that painting to teach - ...it can teach you something about yourself. There is so much going on in the sentence with thinking about the wondering, finding a painting, hearing truisms that create agreement; that to also keep track of the final embedded command is difficult it just sinks in because analysing that as well takes considerable effort.

> D: And there can be something curious about the painting... and as you pay all your attention to me so you can notice the things that I say and the things that I do and perhaps it will be the way that I say things... that's it... and I wonder what it is that's curious about the painting...

I am continuing with many nominalisations and vague phrases like 'curious' 'attention' 'things that I say' 'things that I do' 'way that I say things' 'wonder'. These help to keep the client on an inner search for their own meaning to what I am saying and doing. I sandwich the paying attention to me and emphasising to the client that there is something important in what I am saying and doing between two statements about being curious about the painting. This is partly to create amnesia for this paying attention. I want the client to unconsciously be responsive but to feel these bits haven't been said; that they were just listening to me talking about the painting.

## Open Ended Suggestions

> D: Could it be that movement and I wonder where that movement is and whether it is a little bit of movement or a lot of movement and whether that movement is in the centre or off to the sides or round the edges... and I wonder what type of movement it is whether it's a sort of wavy movement or a swirly movement or some other kind of movement and whether it has a 3d effect or a 2d effect...

While the client is paying attention to the painting I want to generate movement. I don't want to mismatch the client's inner reality (which could include movement or no movement in the painting). I decided to be fairly strong on saying that there is movement so I say there is movement but because I know the client could be seeing a still image I want to cover all bases with suggestions that lead to the movement being their but perhaps not at first observed. I mention the location and give the option for it being a little bit or a lot and the type of movement. I don't want to give a chance for the client to stop and think there is no movement so I say all of these options in fairly quick succession. I'm always implying there is definitely movement there even if at first it was so small it wasn't noticed until I mentioned it.

> D: That's it and you can be curious to *pay attention...* to whether there are sounds there and perhaps they are coming from the picture or from elsewhere and maybe behind you or in front of you or to the left or the right or from above or maybe below... that's it... that's it... that's it...

This is a technique I use quite often; where I will suggest an idea as if any possibility is an option then follow a preferred route. For example, above I suggest paying attention to see if there are sounds there; giving the choice that there may be silence but before the client has time to think about it I suggest that sounds are there it is now a question of where they are coming from. I then go on to give multiple options of where the sounds could be originating.

> D: And another curiosity about this picture is that *you can step inside this picture...* that's

> it... and I don't know what it's like the other side of the picture...

When I said 'step inside the picture' I could see the client had done that by changes in his physiology which I acknowledged by saying 'that's it' I then followed this up by immediately stating a truism that I don't know what it is like the other side of the picture again implying that they do. And for the client to know what it is like they have to be there. By having the client step into the painting, it takes them even deeper into trance. Any time you have someone change where they are in their mind they go deeper and layer their trance experience so that the last place they go gets sandwiched between the previous places, which are sandwiched between the places before that etc... This leads to usually spontaneously getting amnesia for the deeper parts of the trance.

## Metaphors for Unconscious/Conscious Processes

> D: That's it... you know *normally*...that conscious part of you... guides your decisions...guides what you do, what you're thinking about... it's a bit like a driver of a train... the driver is just a small part of the

whole thing... and the driver can just see what is outside his window... and the driver knows that there are 8 carriages behind and the driver knows that each of those carriages is full of people and that each of those people are saying their own things and doing their own things and each of those people are in control of what they're in control of... some are reading newspapers...some are listening to music and some are planning ideas and many of them are lost in thought... that's it... yet all the driver is aware of even though the driver knows all of that is there... is what's through the window...

I have used a metaphor to parallel the conscious mind by having the conscious mind as the driver of a train and the passengers as neurons that are all doing their own thing independent of the driver. People consciously know their mind is doing lots of things at once that they have no awareness of; and that all they are aware of is what they consciously are currently aware of. Like the driver only being able to see out the window. I am conveying this message as a metaphor as this is an easier way to lay down a pattern for the unconscious mind to use.

> D: That's it... whereas the unconscious part of you is like a super being floating above the train like superman flying above the train where he can see the passengers... because he can see through the walls because he can see what they are all doing, he can notice their behaviours their language... he can fly down and talk to them... he can even make them change their behaviours... he can ask someone to stop reading their newspaper and they would stop... he could ask someone to stop listening to music and they would stop... he could interrupt someone having a conversation and they'd forget what it was that they were talking about...

To describe the unconscious mind, I use the term super being as it has many positive connotations; I describe some of the strength of the unconscious mind and what it can influence by talking about how it can influence the passengers. The idea I want to convey is that a conscious knowing and an unconscious doing are two different things. I want the client to be able to 'just do' on an unconscious level.

## Post Hypnotic Suggestion

> D: That's it... now you can be curious... as to how you are going to use all of your unconscious resources... how you are going to use all of the talents you've got that are normally held back behind the doors of the conscious part... you can be curious about what the improvements will be... and how your mind and your circuitry of your brain will make aspects of the improvements permanent in a comfortable way... that's it... that's it... and you can get a sense of what it is like to see you in your mind... to see you in the future...

There is implication running through this section. When you use implication or presuppositions they act like post hypnotic suggestions. By saying 'you are going to' and 'will' it is placing what I am saying in the future as a certainty rather than a possibility. I follow the suggestions up by building on each preceding suggestion; I firstly state what will happen in the future, then I move on to 'see you in your mind' then onto a context for that 'you' that is being seen - in the future. If I didn't add that the client could see themselves at any age and any time even made up ages and times (like in the distant past or a futuristic world). I want to keep what I say as unthreatening as possible so I build one thing on another hoping to go just slightly faster than the client's awareness of what I am suggesting so that I am leading their internal reality now. In the same way that you can wear glasses and not notice until someone mentions them; I want the client to assume they've just not noticed something until I mentioned it; rather than it not previously being a part of their reality.

> D: And you remember Superted... Superted used to say his magic word and he would change from an ordinary teddy bear into a super-teddy bear... and consciously you've watched Superted and you could never quite hear the word...you'd never know consciously what the word is no matter how often you watched it... and you can see yourself... and you can see that you having a code word... and you can watch yourself say that code word to yourself... you can watch yourself say that code word to yourself...

I now use the cartoon character Superted to introduce the idea of a code word for triggering the artistic ability. Ideally, I want the code word to be something internal and unconscious rather than something the client has to consciously say. It is like when a hypnotist sets up the word 'sleep' to re-induce trance. I want the client to have a word to re-induce artistic abilities but I want it to come from the client's unconscious mind. To cement ideas and reprogramming I normally give the idea; then have them watch themselves doing the new behaviour; then have them go into that version of themselves to experience actually doing what they have just watched themselves do. This is generally a very effective way of getting that behaviour into the client's future. It also matches the way people normally do things. They get the information (me giving the idea); then think about what they are going to do (see themselves doing the behaviour); then they do it (stepping into that future them and experiencing it). If you just jump someone into just doing a new behaviour it may not stick because there was no planning or mirroring reality. Also, by doing it this way if there are any problems with the way they see things go it can be changed to be just right before they go into the experience.

> D: And when you watch yourself becoming overwhelmed by that compulsive artistic ability... and I don't know if it's thousands of times or even tens of thousands of times or

even realistic and lifelike... in comparison to how the conscious part of you... that other part of you does art... that's it... that's it... and you can watch and I wonder what you see... and I wonder what you see how well you're doing that art... does it look haphazard to start with like when you watch Rolfe Harris... where that other part... the unconscious part has its own way of drawing where it takes control... *it takes control*... and I wonder whether that you reports that it's like the hand doing all of that work themselves... whether it's like an image just being printed onto a page straight from the mind... whether it's like the hands just get a compulsive feeling... whether it's like the hands get a compulsive feeling to carry out that artistic talent...

People with 'natural' artistic ability or people that are 'naturally' talented at anything generally have a high level of compulsion to do what they are interested in. In this section it is this compulsion that I am working at installing. I offer lots of ideas about how that compulsiveness will take effect and that it comes from the unconscious part of the client not the conscious part. I do this by taking about the hands doing the work and that the unconscious mind has its own drawing style. The presupposition through all of this is still one of that improved drawing ability taking place; it's now a question of what it will be like to the conscious mind as an observer rather than whether it will happen. I am also talking to the client as someone that is still observing that future them. They are not yet in that future them.

> D: And I wonder how long that lasts... is it for 20 minutes or half an hour or is it for a full hour... and I wonder whether it ends because you decide it's time to stop or whether it ends because the time is up... and I wonder how long it lasts... is it twenty minutes, half an hour or maybe even a full hour... or somewhere in-between...

I now limit the duration of that compulsive behaviour. I don't want it to carry on indefinitely because that could have negative effects on work and family life. I want the client's unconscious mind to decide the duration so I offer choices around how long it will last rather than just telling the client how long it will last. Whenever doing any work with clients the therapist needs to be mindful of the positive and negative effects of making the change. By having the client view the changes first it gives them the opportunity to see if the changes are acceptable. If they are not you have given the client the option to decide not to go into themselves when we get to that stage and also to make any changes now before they do. It is a bit like starting with hindsight; the client can see if the changes are acceptable from a dissociated position. Being dissociated gives a useful view on things. Like watching a football match and knowing a player should have passed because you saw another player open; yet the player that should have passed wasn't in a position to see what you could see so made different decisions.

> D: And like all resources... *you can use...* the skills and talents and you can transfer to other areas... and that's TRANCEfer to other areas... that's it... excellent... and you know what it's like to... *step inside that you there and experience that deep compulsive desire to create photorealistic art work...* and I wonder what changes happen at a neurological level that are completely comfortable and healthy that build the talent and increase the talent by temporarily numbing down an area of the

> brain and I wonder how that numbing down takes effect...

I use the term TRANCEfer to imply going into trance to transfer skills and abilities.

### Shutting Down Perceptual Filters

> D: You can be curious as to whether it will be like certain signals not being allowed through or certain signals taking a different route around the brain... performing those talents with those signals taking different route to how you perform it consciously and you can imagine what it is like to be that you there carrying out... that's it... that artistic compulsion... and I wonder what it feels like...do the hands feel tingly... or is it in the arms or is it on the back of the neck...

I want to generate feelings associated with the specific trance of improved artistic ability so I ask what it feels like then I tell the client in the next sentence what it will feel like; that it will be a tingling. I them make the focus on where that tingling will be rather than if there will be a tingling or not. I am also setting up the next part of the session where I want the tingling to be link to energy.

> D: You can be curious as to how that compulsion takes effect once you hear that word and I don't know whether the word is Leonardo, or whether the word is Rafael or some other famous artist... that's it... that's it... that's it... and you can go deeper... and deeper... and you know what somnambulism is... that's right... and when that artistic desire... compulsion takes effect I wonder whether it makes the fingers twitch with nervous energy desperate to carry it out or whether that doesn't show...

The self-hypnotic suggestion is bought back in again here and linked to the feeling/energy. I now make the focus on whether the energy will be visible to others or not rather than if it will be there or not. When I introduce something, I want to be there I like to make the focus on something to do with that new thing rather than if that new thing will be there or not.

> D: And you can imagine in your mind a panel and it's a panel with many levers on... and

> each lever is logically labelled... that's it (he moved)...and you can imagine turning up that lever to artistic ability... putting it up to full... that's it... that's it... and in a moment I'm going to lift up your right hand and when I do I'm not going to tell you to put it down any faster than you... *become absorbed*... in the idea of being a great artist...and I don't know whether it's going to be an artist that is going to be a mixture of many artists or an artist that is going to be greater than any artist you've ever known...that's it... and I don't know whether your hand coming down will take two minutes, three minutes or five minutes or somewhere in between... and I don't know how long that will be on the inside... for you... and I wonder what you get up to while that is happening...

The client already has the experience of using arm movement to go deeper into a trance which is becoming more absorbed. I now use it again to become absorbed in the idea of becoming a great artist. Again, I introduce an idea; the idea of becoming deeper absorbed; then I focus attention on time rather than whether the absorption will happen or not and then change focus to what the conscious mind will be getting up to.

> D: And when it's time to come out of a trance and come all the way back to the room you can come back with the artistic abilities... and I'll let you know when that time is... and I wonder what it will have felt like to have those changes occurred on a deep neurological level... first changes can occur though all the connections, pathways, circuitry... that's it... and on one level when you come back how you can be curious as to where those changes came from and how those changes occurred also...

The suggestions given here are given very directly that when the client comes out of the trance they will come back with the artistic abilities. I use the word occurred rather than occur in the middle of a sentence to imply they have happened; then I mention a curiosity about where those changes have come from to again change the focus from whether it happens or not to trying work out where the changes came from.

D: And I wonder whether you will be amazed or at least shocked... and you know the studies that have been done by shutting down areas temporarily in a healthy way... whether it is shutting down or just not allowing the signals to get through temporarily from the logical rational hemisphere... part of the brain... the creative part of the brain the part that notices fine detail  notices every little thing, notices millions and millions of bits of information every single second... that part of the brain can take control...and then it will end up with you having... (client moved his arm to scratch)... that's it... many abilities... that's it... that's it... now as you're going to achieve great things... that's it... that's it... we want you to take your time to do this... *take your time to do this now...* that's it... that's it... (I lift the clients arm above his head)... that's it... that's it... and on many levels you can begin to count backwards from 100 and let the unconscious work... that's it... and you know what your right foot feels like and I wonder if it feels different from the left... that's it... that's it...

> and your left hand can be left there lightly resting where it is and I wonder how your eyelids feel... that's it...that's it...making this completely...

While the client has their arm in the air and is counting down in his mind I want to jump his attention all over the place to stop him focusing on the lowering arm and the internal unconscious work.

> D: That's it and you know a minute of my time can seem like a longer time of yours just like you can experience... that's it... (arm fully came down)... a longer time that just goes by from minute to minute... and you can take a minute of my time to go deep and comfortable inside your mind into a deep and comfortable focused state of mind... allowing that artistic ability to develop and enhance itself and the more it enhances itself the more pleasure you can experience inside your mind and you can take a minute of total silence to do that now... (minutes silence - I just sit observing minimal cues)...

I sit and observe and watch for signs of increasing pleasure to see that he is enhancing his ability.

> D: That's it... that's it... and you know you can control blood flow, you can make yourself blush on half of your face and if you get a cut you can make it so that the blood stops flowing over the cut any more than is necessary to keep the wound clean... you can make an arm numb or a leg numb or half a head numb... you can increase your metabolism or slow it down... you can alter any system in your body with your mind...

To link back with the earlier statement of making part of the brain numb I sandwich the suggestion for this again in the middle of a collection of truisms about what the mind is capable of.

> D: Now when it's time for you to open your eyes I'll ask you again to draw a horse and again you will get one minute to do it in... and you can be curious as to how much better that horse will be drawn... will it be lifelike, will it be hundreds or thousands of times improved on the last one... how much can you

> manage to draw in one minute…you can be curious as to how much you can draw of that horse in one minute and the level of detail you can draw… and you can always keep in mind that ability those abilities you have… and you can always keep in mind how to get that artistic ability… and you can always keep that in mind… that's it… and you can open your eyes now…

My use of the term 'you can always keep in mind' is specifically used because if you always keep something in mind it means it is always there. It is a post hypnotic suggestion to make everything stick.

> D: (Now talking normally) Right want to have a bash at drawing the horse again… we'll see how it goes now… help if the pen works (pen didn't work so the client changed pen)… (one minute given to re-draw the horse)… times up… how do you think you did?
>
> C: It looks more like a horse than the last one did; it's more proportionate I think
>
> D: Yes, drawing style was different as well
>
> (Client starts to carry on drawing)

C: I'm not supposed to be doing this now am I?

D: No, I'll show this to the camera before we... if you do start finishing it off or something

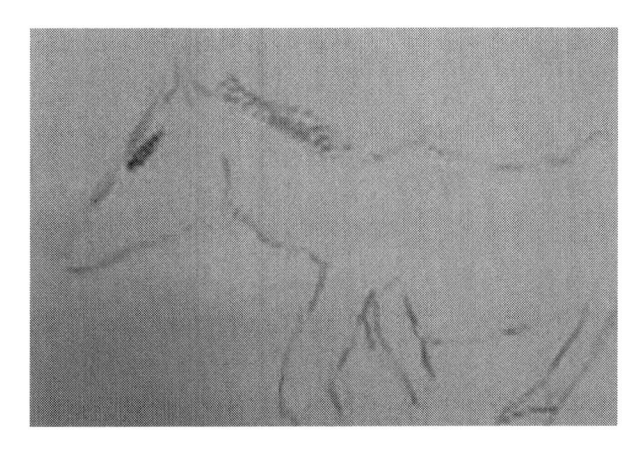

C: That is quite different isn't it (client picks up a pen again to carry on drawing)

D: And that's only a first thing drawn after being zapped

Next few minutes was spent me just watching as the client compulsively kept drawing, putting the pen down to talk then carrying on getting absorbed in drawing again, getting more involved in what he was doing and adding more and more detail, then adding colour and motion. In total he spent about 4 minutes on the picture adding to it, putting the pen down for a few moments to talk but then not talking instead he would pick the pen up and carry on drawing. I tried to get his attention to discuss his experience but he struggled to tell me as he was more absorbed in continuing to draw. Below is the picture after about four minutes of drawing on it.

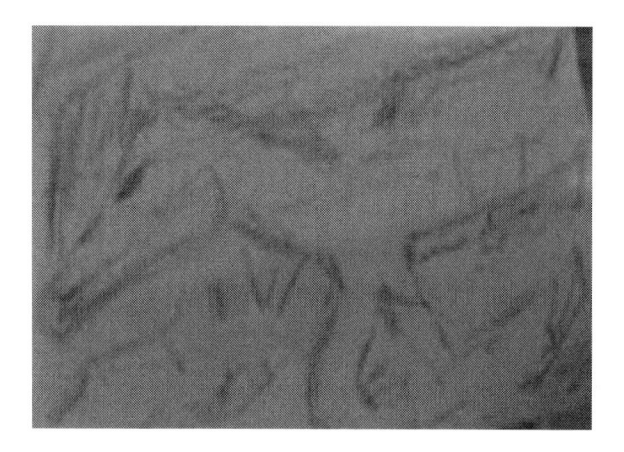

After the session the client went home and drew an image off of a Disney video case. He said it only took him a few minutes to sketch it. He then put it on his computer and coloured it in. He said he was amazed at what he had done and didn't understand how it was possible. Since then he continued to draw in this new way and felt compelled to draw and has since gone on to teach himself to play guitar and piano and other creative pursuits.

# Conclusion

This book is the second in a planned series of ten books on hypnotherapy. In this book I have shared my perspective of the Ericksonian approach. If you take the time to learn and master the content in the book you will be way ahead of many other therapists in your ability to help people. You will be able to do hypnosis without the need for rigid hypnotherapy scripts. You will be client-centred and able to be responsive to the needs of your clients and you will be able to be creative in your interventions. Book three *Hypnotherapy Revealed: Hypnotherapy Trance Scripts* will share a wide selection of hypnotic induction and therapeutic scripts as well as additional information about how using the hypnosis scripts fits within therapy, how to structure therapy sessions and how to understand and use the scripts. This book and the *Introduction to Hypnotherapy* book came first because I wouldn't want someone reading *Hypnotherapy Trance Scripts* and becoming a hypnotherapist who just reads scripts. I want the readers of that book to be comfortable to work unscripted who will use the scripts for ideas and for education.

Until next time

Dan Jones

# BIBLIOGRAPHY

Alpert, J. (2012, April 21). *In Therapy Forever?* Retrieved from The New York Times: https://www.nytimes.com/2012/04/22/opinion/sunday/in-therapy-forever-enough-already.html

Andrillon, T., Nir, Y., Cirelli, C., Tononi, G., & Fried, I. (2015). Single-neuron activity and eye movements during human REM sleep and awake vision. *Nature Communications, 6*(7884).

Atkinson, D., Rossi, E., Rossi, K., Hill, R., Iannotti, S., Cozzolino, M., . . . Kerouac, M. (2010). A New Bioinformatics Paradigm for the Theory, Research, and Practice of Therapeutic Hypnosis. *53*(1).

Barbar, T. X. (1981). *Hypnosis: a scientific approach.* Power Publishers Inc.

Bargh, J. A., & Chartrand, T. L. (2000). The mind in the middle: A practical guide to priming and automaticity research. In H. T. Reis, & C. M. Judd, *Handbook of research methods in social and personality psychology* (pp. 253-285). New York: Cambridge University Press.

Bargh, J. A., & Morsella, E. (2008). The Unconscious Mind. *Perspectives on Psychological Science, 3*(1).

Bargh, J. A., & Morsella, E. (2010). Unconscious Behavioral Guidance Systems. In C. R. Agnew, D. E. Carlston, & W. G. Graziano, *Then a Miracle Occurs: Focusing on Behavior in Social Psychological Theory and Research* (pp. 89-118). Oxford: Oxford University Press.

Baumeister, R. F., DeWall, C. N., Vohs, K. D., & Alquist, J. L. (2010). Does Emotion Cause Behavior (Apart from Making People Do Stupid, Destructive Things)? In C.

R. Agnew, D. E. Carlston, W. G. Graziano, & J. R. Kelly, *Then A Miracle Occurs.* Oxford: Oxford University Press.

BBC. (2010). *Horizon: Is Seeing Believing? The McGurk Effect.* Retrieved from YouTube: https://youtu.be/G-lN8vWm3m0

Bell, D. R. (2013). Integrative Functions of the Central Nervous System. In R. A. Rhoades, & D. R. Bell, *Medical Physiology: Principles for Clinical Medicine (4th Edition)* (p. 119). Lippincott Williams & Wilkins.

Berger, J., Meredith, M., & Wheeler, S. C. (2008). Contextual priming: Where people vote affects how they vote. *Proceedings of the National Academy of Sciences of the United States of America, 105*(26).

Broom, B. (2002). Somatic Metaphors: a clinical phenomenon pointing to a new model of disease, personhood, and physical reality. *18*(1).

Brown, R. E., Basheer, R., McKenna, J. T., Strecker, R. E., & McCarley, R. W. (2012). Control of Sleep and Wakefulness. *Physiology Review, 92*.

Burlingame, C. C. (1947). Psychosomatic Elements: When The Foreman is a Pain in the Neck. *11*(3).

Caine, R. N., & Caine, G. (1991). *Making Connections: Teaching and the Human Brain.* Association for Supervision and Curriculum Development.

Callaway, C. W., Lydic, R., Baghdoyan, H. A., & Hobson, J. (1987). Pontogeniculooccipital waves: spontaneous visual system activity during rapid eye movement sleep. *Cellular and Molecular Neurobiology, 7*(2).

Carr, M., & Nielsen, T. A. (2015). Daydreams and Nap Dreams: Content Comparisons. *Consciousness and Cognition, 36*.

Christoff, K., Gordon, A. M., Smallwood, J., Smith, R., & Schooler, J. W. (2009). Experience sampling during fMRI reveals default network and executive system contributions to mind wandering. *Proceedings of the National Academy of Sciences, 106*(21).

Clark, G. A. (1995). Emotional Learning: Fear and loathing in the amygdala. *Current Biology, 5*(3).

Cozzolino, M., Iannotti, S., Castiglione, S., Cicatelli, A., Rossi, K., & Rossi, E. (2014). A bioinformatic analysis of the molecular-genomic signature of therapeutic hypnosis. *The International Journal of Psychosocial and Cultural Genomics, 1*(1).

Csikszentmihalyi, M. (1990). *Flow: The psychology of optimal experience.* New York: Harper & Row.

Diamond, M. J. (1987). The Interactional Basis of Hypnotic Experience: On the Relational Dimensions of Hypnosis. *International Journal of Clinical and Experimental Hypnosis, 35*(2).

Ellenberger, H. F. (1970). *The Discovery of the Unconscious.* Basic Books.

Elman, L. (2016). *The History of Dave Elman and the D.E.H.I.* Retrieved from Dave Elman Hypnosis Institute: www.elmanhypnosis.com/history

Erickson, B., & Keeney, B. P. (2006). *Milton H. Erickson, M.D.: An American Healer.* Carmarthen: Crown House Publishing.

Erickson, M. H. (1932). Possible Detrimental Effects Of Experimental Hypnosis. *The Journal of Abnormal and Social Psychology, 27*(3).

Erickson, M. H. (1952). Deep Hypnosis and Its Induction. In L. M. LeCron, *Experimental Hypnosis.* New York: Macmillan.

Erickson, M. H. (1964). Initial Experiments Investigating the Nature of Hypnosis. *The American Journal of Clinical Hypnosis, 7*(2).

Erickson, M. H. (1964). The "Surprise" and "My-Friend-John" Techniques of Hypnosis: Minimal Cues and Natural

Field Experimentation. *The American Journal of Clinical Hypnosis, 6*(4).

Erickson, M. H. (1964). The Confusion Technique in Hypnosis. *The American Journal of Clinical Hypnosis, 6*(3).

Erickson, M. H. (1977). The Control of Physiological Functions by Hypnosis. *The American Journal of Clinical Hypnosis, 20*(1).

Erickson, M. H. (1980). Explorations in Hypnosis Research. In M. H. Erickson, & E. L. Rossi, *The Collected Papers of Milton H Erickson on Hypnosis Volume 2: Hypnotic Alteration of Sensory, Perceptual and Psychophysiological Processes.* New York: Irvington Publishers Inc.

Erickson, M. H. (1980). Hypnotic Alteration of Blood Flow: An Experiment Comparing Waking and Hypnotic Responsiveness. In M. H. Erickson, & E. L. Rossi, *The Collected Papers of Milton H Erickson on Hypnosis Volume 2: Hypnotic alteration of sensory, perceptual and psychophysical processes.* New York: Irvington Publishers Inc.

Erickson, M. H. (2008). Respiratory Rhythm in Trance Induction: The Role of Minimal Sensory Cues in Normal and Trance Behavior. In E. L. Rossi, R. Erickson-Klein, & K. L. Rossi, *The Collected Works of Milton H Erickson: Volume 1: The Nature of Therapeutic Hypnosis* (pp. 307-312). Phoenix: The Milton Erickson Foundation.

Erickson, M. H., & Rossi, E. L. (1976). *Hypnotic Realities.* Irvington Publishers Inc.

Erickson, M. H., & Rossi, E. L. (1976). The Indirect Forms of Suggestion. In M. H. Erickson, & E. L. Rossi, *Collected Papers of Milton H Erickson* (Vol. 4). New York: Irvington Publishers Inc.

Erickson, M. H., & Rossi, E. L. (1977). Autohypnotic Experiences of Milton H. Erickson. *The American Journal of Clinical Hypnosis, 20*(1).

Erickson, M. H., & Rossi, E. L. (1981). *Experiencing Hypnosis: Therapeutic Approaches to Altered States.* New York: Irvington Publishers Inc.

Forrest, D. (2000). *Hypnotism: A History.* London: Penguin Group.

Gilligan, S. (1982). Ericksonian Approaches To Clinical Hypnosis. In J. K. Zeig, *Ericksonian Approaches to Hypnosis and Psychotherapy.* New York: Brunner/Mazel.

Gollwitzer, P. M., Wieber, F., Myers, A. L., & McCrea, S. M. (2010). How to Maximise Implementation Intention Effects. In C. R. Agnew, D. E. Carlston, G. W. G, & J. R. Kelly, *The a Miracle Occurs.* Oxford: Oxford University Press.

Gorder, P. F. (2018, March 19). *At first blush, you look happy - or sad, or angry.* Retrieved from The Ohio State University: https://news.osu.edu/news/2018/03/19/firstblush/

Grecco, E., Robbins, S. J., Bartoli, E., & Wolff, E. F. (2013). Use of Nonconscious Priming to Promote Self-Disclosure. *Clinical Psychological Science, 1*(3).

Griffin, J. (2006). Molar Memories: how an ancient mechanism can ruin lives. *Human Givens Journal, 13*(3).

Griffin, J. (2007). *The Expectation Fulfilment Theory Of Dreaming.* Retrieved from Why We Dream: https://www.why-we-dream.com/thetheory.htm

Griffin, J. (2012). *7-11 breathing: How does deep breathing make you feel more relaxed?* Retrieved from The Human Givens Institute: https://www.hgi.org.uk/resources/delve-our-extensive-library/resources-and-techniques/7-11-breathing-how-does-deep

Griffith, F. L., & Thompson, H. (1904). *The Demotic Magical Papyrus of London and Leiden.* London: H. Grevel & Co. Retrieved from Sacred Texts: http://www.sacred-texts.com/egy/dmp/

Guy, K., & Guy, N. (2003). The fast cure for phobia and trauma: evidence that it works. *Human Givens Journal, 9*(4).

Heap, M. (2017). Theories of Hypnosis. In G. Elkins, *Handbook of Medical and Psychological Hypnosis.* New York: Springer Publishing Company LLC.

Hoeft, F., Gabrieli, J. D., Whitfield-Gabrieli, S., Haas, B. W., Bammer, R., Menon, V., & Spiegel, D. (2012). Functional Brain Basis of Hypnotizability. *Archives of General Psychiatry, 69*(10).

Hull, C. (2002). *Hypnosis and Suggestibility.* Carmarthen: Crown House Publishing.

Jiang, H., White, M. P., Greicius, M. D., Waelde, L. C., & Spiegel, D. (2017). Brain Activity and Functional Connectivity Associated with Hypnosis. *Cerebral Cortex, 27*(8).

Kincaid, J. C. (2013). Autonomic Nervous System. In R. A. Rhoades, & D. R. Bell, *Medical Physiology: Principles for Clinical Medicine (4th Edition)* (p. 114). Lippincott Williams & Wilkins.

Kirsch, I., Montgomery, G., & Sapirstein, G. (1995). Hypnosis as an Adjunct to Cognitive-Behavioral Psychotherapy: A Meta-Analysis. *63*(2).

Kleitman, N. (1982). Basic Rest-Activity Cycle—22 Years Later. *Sleep, 5*(4).

Krueger, J. (2015). *Flow and Happiness: Do you have to be an expert to be happy?* Retrieved from Psychology Today:

https://www.psychologytoday.com/us/blog/one-among-many/201502/flow-and-happiness

Lally, P., Van Jaarsveld, C. H., Potts, H. W., & Wardle, J. (2010). How are habits formed: Modelling habit formation in the real world. *40*(6).

Lankton, S. R., & Lankton, C. H. (1983). *The Answer Within: A Clinical Framework of Ericksonian Hypnotherapy.* New York: Brunner/Mazel.

Larkin, W. K. (2011, September 26). *Thoughts or Feelings? Which Comes First?* Retrieved from The Applied Neuroscience Blog: http://appliedneuroscienceblog.com/thoughts_or_feelings_which_comes_first

Latham, G., & Shantz, A. (2011). The effect of primed goals on employee performance: Implications for human resource management. *Human Resource Management, 50*(2).

Lehmann, M., Schreiner, T., Rasch, B., & Seifritz, E. (2016). Emotional arousal modulates oscillatory correlates of targeted memory reactivation during NREM, but not REM sleep. *Scientific Reports*(39229).

Lustig, H. L. (1988). So Whose Therapy Am I Using Anyhow? In J. K. Zeig, & S. R. Lankton, *Developing Ericksonian Therapy: A State of the Art.* Bristol, Pennsylvania: Brunner/Mazel.

Lynn, S. J., Green, J. P., Weekes, J. R., Carlson, B. W., Brentar, J., Latham, L., & Kurzhals, R. (1990). Literalism and Hypnosis: Hypnotic versus Task-Motivated Subjects. *American Journal of Clinical Hypnosis, 33*(2).

Lynn, S. J., Laurence, J.-R., & Kirsch, I. (2015). Hypnosis, Suggestion, and Suggestibility:An Integrative Model. *American Journal of Clinical Hypnosis, 57*(3).

Marchese, M. H., Robbins, S. J., & Morrow, M. T. (2018). Nonconscious priming enhances the therapy relationship: An experimental analog study. *Psychotherapy Research, 28*(2).

Matthews, W. J., Conti, J., & Starr, L. (1999). Ericksonian Hypnosis: A Review Of the Empirical Data. *Sleep and Hypnosis, 1*(1).

Merikle, D. M. (1988). Subliminal auditory messages: An evaluation. *Psychology Marketing, 5*, 355-372.

Moll, A. (1890). *Hypnotism*. London: Walter Scott.

Montgomery, G. H., Schnur, J. B., & David, D. (2011). The impact of hypnotic suggestibility in clinical care settings. *International Journal of Clinical and Experimental Hypnosis, 59*(3).

Morgan, A. H., & Hilgard, E. R. (1973). Age differences in susceptibility to hypnosis. *International Journal of Clinical and Experimental Hypnosis, 21*(2).

Morgan, A. H., Johnson, D. L., & Hilgard, E. R. (1974). The stability of hypnotic susceptibility: A longitudinal study. *International Journal of Clinical and Experimental Hypnosis, 22*(3).

Morrison, A. R. (1999). A Scientist at Work: Exploring the Neurobiology of Sleep. *The American Biology Teacher, 61*(7).

Pace-Schott, E. F. (2003). Postscript: Recent findings on the neurobiology of sleep and dreaming. In E. F. Pace-Schott, M. Solms, M. Blagrove, & S. Harnad, *Sleep and Dreaming: Scientific Advances and Reconsiderations.* Cambridge: Cambridge University Press.

Page, R. A., & Green, J. P. (2007). An Update on Age, Hypnotic Suggestibility, and Gender: A Brief Report. *The American Journal of Clinical Hypnosis, 49*(4).

Parsons-Fein, J. A. (2013). *In The Room With Milton H Erickson.* Parsons-Fein Press.

Pintar, J., & Lynn, S. J. (2008). *Hypnosis: A Brief History.* Chichester: John Wiley & Sons.

Queensland Brain Institute. (n.d.). *What Makes Memories Stronger?* Retrieved from The University of Queensland, Australia: https://qbi.uq.edu.au/brain-basics/memory/what-makes-memories-stronger

Rasch, B., & Born, J. (2013). About Sleep's Role in Memory. *Physiological Reviews, 93*(2).

Rosen, S. (1991). *My Voice Will Go With You: The Teaching Tales of Milton H Erickson MD.* New York: W W Norton & Company.

Salamone, J. D., & Correa, M. (2012). The Mysterious Motivational Functions of Mesolimbic Dopamine. *Neuron, 76*(3). Retrieved from Cell.com: https://www.cell.com/neuron/fulltext/S0896-6273(12)00941-5

Sanford, L. D., Tejani-Butt, S. M., Ross, R. J., & Morrison, A. R. (1996). Amygdaloid Control of Alerting and Behavioural Arousal in Rats: Involvement of Serotonergic Mechanisms. *Archives Italiennes de Biologie: A Journal of Neuroscience, 134*(1).

Schafer, S. M., Colloca, L., & Wager, T. D. (2015). Conditioned Placebo Analgesia Persists When Subjects Know They Are Receiving a Placebo. *The Journal of Pain, 16*(5).

Short, D. (2017). *Principles and Core Competencies of Ericksonian Therapy: The 2017 Research and Teaching Manual for Ericksonian Therapy.* Phoenix: The Milton H Erickson Foundation.

Sidis, B. (1898). *The Psychology of Suggestion.* New York: Appleton.

Snyder, A. (2009). Explaining and inducing savant skills: privileged access to lower level, less-processed information. *Philosophical Transactions of the Royal Society*(364), 1399-1405.

Stickgold, R. (2002). EMDR: A Putative Neurobiological Mechanism of Action. *JOURNAL OF CLINICAL PSYCHOLOGY, 58*(1).

Tyrrell, M. (2015). *The Most Important Psychological Insight I Ever Learnt*. Retrieved from Uncommon Knowledge: https://www.unk.com/blog/most-important-psychological-insight-ever-learnt/

Vyazovskiy, V. V., & Delogu, A. (2014). NREM and REM Sleep: Complementary Roles in Recovery after Wakefulness. *The Neuroscientist, 20*(3).

Waterfield, R. (2002). *Hidden Depths*. London: Macmillan.

Welch, M. G. (2017). *Family Nurture Intervention*. Retrieved from Nurture Science Program, Columbia University Medical Center: https://nurturescienceprogram.org/family-nurture-intervention/

Werrell, B. (2013). *Why Daydreaming is an Essential Part of Learning*. Retrieved from Connections Academy: http://blog.connectionsacademy.com/why-daydreaming-is-an-essential-part-of-learning/

*What is Ericksonian Hypnosis and What Characterizes It*. (n.d.). Retrieved from Natural Hypnosis: https://www.naturalhypnosis.com/blog/what-is-ericksonian-hypnosis-and-how-is-it-used

*What is Ericksonian Hypnosis? Definition & History*. (n.d.). Retrieved from British Hypnosis Research: https://britishhypnosisresearch.com/about-ericksonian-hypnotherapy/

Williams, L. E., & Bargh, J. A. (2008). Experiencing Physical Warmth Promotes Interpersonal Warmth. *322*(5901).

Zeig, J. (1977). Symptom Prescription and Ericksonian Principles of Hypnosis and Psychotherapy. *20th Annual Scientific Meeting of the American Society of*

*Clinical Hypnosis.* Atlanta, Georgia: American Society of Clinical Hypnosis.

Zeig, J. (1980). *A Teaching Seminar With Milton H Erickson.* New York: Brunner Mazel.

Zeig, J. (1999). The Virtues of Our Faults: A key concept of Ericksonian therapy. *1*(2).

Zeig, J. (2014). *The Induction of Hypnosis.* Phoenix, Arizona: Milton H Erickson Foundation Press.